NEUROPATHY

HOW TO RELIEVE FOOT NUMBNESS,TINGLING, BURNING, AND CRAMPING WITHOUT DRUGS OR SURGERY

DR. PHILIP A STRAW D.C.

ISBN: 1492148482
ISBN 13: 9781492148487

Library of Congress Control Number: 2013915567
CreateSpace Independent Publishing Platform
North Charleston, South Carolina

TABLE OF CONTENTS

INTRODUCTION

If you're reading this book, the chances are that you or a loved one has been diagnosed with peripheral neuropathy. Or perhaps you are experiencing numbness or pain in your toes or feet and you want to learn more about what might be at the core of the problem. This book is here to help.

My goal is to give you the most important tool you will ever receive regarding peripheral neuropathy—and that is useful information. With the right information, you'll be able to make the kind of health and treatment choices that will, in short, transform your life or the life of a loved one.

Right now you might be living with the notion that there is nothing you or your doctor can do about peripheral neuropathy, but that really isn't the case. We will explore steps that you can take to dramatically reduce your peripheral-neuropathy pain.

Seven Key Questions We Will Explore in this Book

1. What is peripheral neuropathy?
2. What causes peripheral neuropathy?
3. What are my treatment options?
4. What steps should I be taking to reduce my symptoms?
5. Where should I go for help?
6. What should I really expect from a health-care provider treating my peripheral neuropathy?
7. How can my diet help my neuropathy?

As we begin this journey together to learn about peripheral neuropathy and the different treatments available for patients, I first want to give you a little background about how I got to the point of writing this book today. I've been an alternative health-care professional since 1997. Originally, I was trained as a chiropractor, and I received my doctor of chiropractic degree in 1995.

Initially, as I started in practice, my goal was to help people regain their health without prescription drugs and surgical interventions. I worked in a multidisciplinary practice, and our common goal was to help patients relieve chronic pain, increase function, improve quality of life, and eliminate the need for prescription pain medications and surgical intervention. Quite frequently, patients on multiple prescription pain medications would come to our practice.

Primary physicians told these patients that, other than taking medication, there was nothing else that could be done for their peripheral-neuropathy pain and that they would have to "live with it." I summarily rejected this notion and sought to find a better option.

In 2001, I started a complementary alternative-medicine (CAM) practice. I call this practice *alternative*. However, if you are familiar with statistics at all, you already know that more people are seeking alternative health care than at any time in history. Total office visits to alternative providers are, in fact, outpacing the number of patients going to primary doctors.

People's awareness level is being raised to the point where they only want to take prescription drugs or consider surgery as a last resort. **Increasingly, patients are realizing that most prescription medications don't treat the cause; they just mask the symptoms.**

In 2006, I had a new patient who would change everything.

MY EXPERIENCE WITH LAUREN

Lauren was in her thirties and came to our practice seeking help for her chronic pain. She was the mother of two boys under the age of five. Lauren had been taking five Vicodin a day just to function and get through the daily grind.

Lauren had already undergone two failed surgeries. She had chronic nerve damage and pain in her leg and back. I mention her case because it was a turning point in my practice. We'd been able to tackle most patients' problems and help them get off medications and even avoid surgery.

First we put Lauren through our traditional protocols. I'd like to tell you she was off Vicodin after six weeks of care, but she was still taking five a day. In short, we failed her.

This motivated me to keep researching what else was out there. I wanted to find a different approach so that people like Lauren could find relief. I knew that there had to be a different way. What other technologies were out there? I went on a quest for answers.

I pored over research, investigated, and probed. It kept me up at night and became an obsession. Eventually the answer did come. Just six months after I failed to help Lauren, I invested $250,000 on new technology for chronic pain.

I immediately called Lauren. She was still in the same amount of pain— maybe even a little bit more. I invited her to come back into the office, putting her through my updated protocols with the new technologies I had installed. I was very encouraged when she responded favorably. Lauren was getting better, and the pain that was sucking the life out of her was finally going away.

Within two weeks, she was off almost all of her Vicodin. After six weeks, she was 95 percent free of chronic pain. About three months after she started treatment, she was leading a healthy, normal, pain-free life taking care of her young family. The new approach had worked.

Working with Lauren was a real turning point for me. I'll never forget her. I realized that there is always an answer out there. If you don't have it, you have to keep looking until you find it.

In the course of living our daily lives, it is difficult for most of us to realize just how fast technology is moving. This rapid technological evolution isn't just occurring in the realm of electronics and computers. Computers speed is doubled every twenty-four months, and we are seeing similar accelerated change in areas like biotechnology and medical technology. We should expect to see a wide array of advancements across the health-care spectrum in the coming years. These advancements will not be limited to pharmaceuticals alone.

By seeking out these advancements, you can dramatically improve your health and address your peripheral-neuropathy pain. This book is about helping you learn more about these advancements. I'll reveal the latest and most effective alternative treatments that are specifically geared toward addressing peripheral-neuropathy pain. Technology and medicine are changing quickly, and this fact holds true for peripheral-neuropathy treatment as well.

Fast-forward from 2006 to 2014. My practice has evolved to where I only help patients with peripheral neuropathy. Today 100 percent of my practices are focused on using new and clinically proven technologies, the latest research, and the most up-to-date understanding of nutrition to help patients with peripheral neuropathy.

By reading this book, you're going to learn exactly what peripheral neuropathy is and what it's not. We'll explore the causes and learn

TRY THIS FOR SLEEPING

ALMOND MILK
TURMERIC   FOR
CINNAMON   SLEEPING

...MATION DISTRIBUTION PROJECT
...L PROJECT OF
...TY GUARD
...Box 1645
...VA 22116-1645

THE FINISH PEOPLE STOP
PUTTING BUTTER ON EVERYTHING THEY ATE.
CUT THE SATURATED FAT AND LOTS OF THE
RED MEAT. BEGAN EATING MORE FRUITS &
VEGETABLES.

more about your options. As you will discover, your options are in no way limited to a life of taking pills and living with the misery of numbness and pain in your feet.

The notion that peripheral neuropathy is destined to rob you of your mobility and the ability to enjoy your retirement years is an antiquated idea.

Now, let's turn our attention to the options that you have and how these options can and will change your life.

PART ONE

CAUSES, DIAGNOSIS, AND TREATMENT OF PERIPHERAL NEUROPATHY

CHAPTER ONE

WHAT IS PERIPHERAL NEUROPATHY?

If you or someone you love has peripheral neuropathy, there is hope. Here we will explore this condition and what you can do to treat it. With knowledge, it is possible for you to effectively improve your condition. Like so much in life, the first and most important step is to gain the right information so that you can make informed decisions that lead to the best possible outcomes.

A key part of addressing your peripheral neuropathy or helping someone you know with this condition is to understand it. The fact is that twenty million people suffer from this condition—and that is just in the United States. With numbers of this magnitude, it is, of course, rather shocking that you don't hear more about peripheral neuropathy, its causes, and how it can be treated.

While not a household word, peripheral neuropathy is, indeed, very common. In fact, this issue is particularly common in the senior community, and it is estimated that **peripheral neuropathy will affect between 25 and 30 percent of Americans at some point in their lives**.

When an individual has nerve damage or nerve dysfunction in the peripheral nervous system, then he or she has peripheral neuropathy and experiences the accompanying symptoms. A simple look at the nervous system itself will help in understanding more about this condition. Let's take a closer look.

THE TWO KEY PARTS OF YOUR NERVOUS SYSTEM

The nervous system is broken up into two major parts: the central nervous system, which consists of your brain and spinal cord, and your peripheral nervous system, which is composed of all the nerves that go from your spinal cord to your arms, legs, and internal organs.

Sensory nerves are part of the peripheral nervous system. These nerves provide sensory information directly to your brain from your environment. An example of how this works would be your experience if you touched a hot stove. This would result in the sensory nerves in your hand sending a signal to your brain, alerting you that the surface is hot and dangerous.

The brain very quickly responds by sending a signal down your motor nerves to your hand. In the process, your muscles contract so you quickly move your hands away from the hot stove. In the case of healthy nerves, this whole process happens in just a nanosecond.

However, for those with peripheral neuropathy, the story is quite different. If you have peripheral neuropathy in your feet and you step barefoot on hot sand in the middle of summer, you might not feel it. Your brain doesn't get the signal from the damaged nerves in your feet, and you end up with third-degree burns. As you can imagine, the health and safety implications of peripheral neuropathy are nothing short of tremendous. Living with this issue is dangerous and quite serious. Peripheral neuropathy warrants attention and treatment.

WHAT'S NEUROPATHY

The term "neuropathy" refers to any disease that impacts the nervous system and its neurons. Your nerves are an essential part of your body, as they provide essential communication. If the nerves are damaged, they will no longer be able to function properly.

Depending on how many and what nerves are affected by neuropathy, different issues will result. For example, if just one nerve is damaged, a patient will suffer from a condition called mononeuropathy; if several nerves are impacted, polyneuropathy will result.

The peripheral nervous system consists of sensory nerves, motor nerves, and autonomic nerves

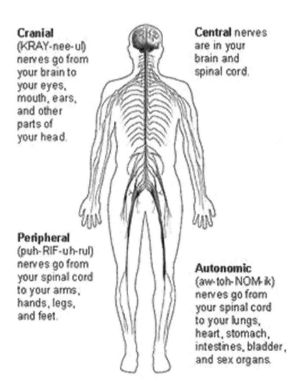

Cranial (KRAY-nee-ul) nerves go from your brain to your eyes, mouth, ears, and other parts of your head.

Central nerves are in your brain and spinal cord.

Peripheral (puh-RIF-uh-rul) nerves go from your spinal cord to your arms, hands, legs, and feet.

Autonomic (aw-toh-NOM-ik) nerves go from your spinal cord to your lungs, heart, stomach, intestines, bladder, and sex organs.

Your peripheral nervous system actually contains all nerves, except those within the brain and the spinal cord. However, the peripheral nervous system does transmit information from the brain and spinal cord throughout the body. As a result, those with peripheral neuropathy experience varied symptoms from head to toe. Researchers have currently identified more than one hundred kinds of peripheral neuropathy.

THE AUTONOMIC NERVOUS SYSTEM

The autonomic nervous system controls all the parts of your body that are essentially on autopilot. These are the body functions that you do not have to actively think about in order to function and live, such as your heartbeat, breathing, digestive system, and circulatory system.

There is also a condition called autonomic neuropathy, which impacts bodily functions that you can't control. With this issue, your heart rate, sweating, blood pressure, and digestion are impacted.

Those with autonomic neuropathy will suffer from symptoms, such as dizziness, shakiness, sweating, heart palpitations, urination malfunction, sexual issues, digestive problems, cardiovascular issues, and even the inability to exercise. Again, autonomic neuropathy is a very different condition. To summarize, it is the result of damage to the nerves that regulate functions of the body that aren't actively controlled.

WHAT ARE THE SYMPTOMS OF PERIPHERAL NEUROPATHY?

Considering the health and safety hazards that peripheral neuropathy represents, it is essential to understand its symptoms. Once you understand the various symptoms associated with peripheral neuropathy, you will be able to decide whether or not you or a loved one should seek out medical attention.

Three Key Peripheral-Neuropathy Symptom Facts

1. The symptoms of peripheral neuropathy are caused by nerve damage.
2. The symptoms vary, depending on the type and location of the nerves involved.
3. The most common symptoms of peripheral neuropathy happen in the feet and sometimes the hands. Typically, but not always, patients first notice symptoms in the toes or balls of their feet.

Peripheral Neuropathy Symptoms Can Include

1. Tingling
2. Numbness
3. Changes in sensation
4. On occasion, severe pain at night
5. Burning sensations
6. An inability to sense hot and/or cold
7. Loss of coordination
8. Loss of dexterity
9. Inability to feel clothing, such as socks or gloves
10. Muscle weakness
11. Difficulty walking
12. Muscle twitching
13. Muscle cramps
14. Leg spasms
15. Loss of muscle control
16. Falling and increased risk of falling
17. In the most severe cases, it is even possible to lose the ability to move parts of the body

THE TYPE 2 DIABETES

Currently the Western world is experiencing a serious and unprecedented increase in obesity and type 2 diabetes. In a statistic that is shocking and revealing, an incredible 60 to 70 percent of those with diabetes will also develop peripheral neuropathy.

Type 2 diabetics have several mechanisms that cause peripheral neuropathy. The first factor is high blood-sugar levels. High blood sugar causes high osmotic pressure in the nerve cells. This, in turn, damages nerves and causes oxidative stress within the nerve cells.

According to the Centers for Disease Control (CDC), one out of ten adults have diabetes. By 2050, the CDC projects that this number will skyrocket to one out of three adults. Simply stated, diabetes dramatically increases one's risk of developing peripheral neuropathy. Looking at the statistics, it is clear that, in the future, more and more people will suffer from peripheral neuropathy.

Although it happens on some occasions, it's not very common for people under fifty to develop peripheral neuropathy. The majority of peripheral neuropathy cases occur among patients that are retired and in their late sixties, seventies, or eighties.

MICROVASCULAR DISEASE

Type 2 diabetes causes microvascular disease, as nerves are dependent on good levels of blood flow to bring them the oxygen they need to function properly. What is microvascular disease? Microvascular disease occurs when tiny blood vessels, called capillaries, become damaged from high blood sugar. High blood sugar results in inflammation, which, in turn, leads to damaged blood vessels and microvascular disease. If you are thinking that microvascular disease sounds destructive, you are, of course, right.

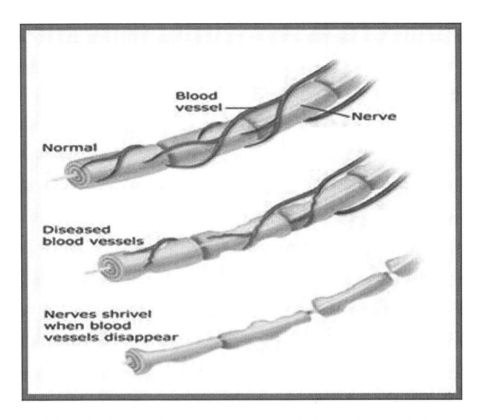

High blood sugar decreases the amount of nitric oxide the body produces. Why is this important for your health? Nitric oxide makes blood vessels open up wider (this is called vasodilation), and in the process, it increases blood flow to the nerves. If nitric oxide levels become too low in the blood vessels, they cause the blood vessels to constrict and decrease blood flow. This leads to hypoxia (decreased oxygen), which leads to nerve damage.

TYPE 2 DIABETES AND GLUTATHIONE, THE MOTHER OF ALL ANTIOXIDANTS

In this book, we will be discussing the role glutathione has in maintaining your health. You've likely heard about the importance of antioxidants and making sure that you get enough in your diet, but what you may not have heard about is the tremendous importance of glutathione.

Type 2 diabetes decreases the level of glutathione in the body. Glutathione is considered the mother of all antioxidants and is made in your body; however, with chronic diseases like diabetes, glutathione levels in the body become depleted. This leads to massive free-radical damage to your nerves. Clearly, glutathione is essential for good health.

We will discuss how you can make sure to maintain optimum glutathione levels.

Some patients ask, "I'm not a diabetic, so what's causing my peripheral neuropathy?" The answer is prediabetes.

Some health statistics can be pretty shocking, and here is one of them: the CDC estimates that 79 million people in America are prediabetic. Prediabetes is a condition of elevated blood sugar that often leads to type 2 diabetes—usually within a few years.

The American Diabetes Association defines a normal fasting blood glucose as less than one hundred mg/dL. Today we consider fasting blood sugars of 100 mg/dL to 125 mg/dL to be prediabetic. The diagnosis of diabetes is made when blood sugar reaches 126 mg/dL or higher.

In my practice, I routinely find patients who are prediabetic and don't even know it. Most patients don't understand that it is possible to start developing peripheral neuropathy even if not technically a diabetic. Prediabetes is the cause of peripheral neuropathy in over 20 percent of my patients. So if you're wondering if your neuropathy is being caused by prediabetes, get your blood sugar tested. If your fasting glucose is over 100 mg/dL but below 125 mg/dL, then you have prediabetes.

CHOLESTEROL MEDICATION

In what is a true shock for most people, taking cholesterol medication can cause peripheral neuropathy. Perhaps even more shocking is the fact that most doctors are not aware of the connection between cholesterol medication and peripheral neuropathy.

In the United States, we continue to spend more and more on statins to lower cholesterol. In 2010, spending increased by $160 million, to almost $19 billion, according to the IMS Institute for Healthcare Informatics. That's over 255 million prescriptions for these drugs in 2010, making them the most commonly prescribed type of medication in the United States.

Our health system believes that prescribing statin medication is the best way to protect your heart. Unfortunately, the link between cholesterol medication and peripheral neuropathy is enough to ask, "Is this the best solution?"

The medical community is placing nearly every senior on these drugs. Yet, even with most seniors taking statins, heart disease is still the nation's number-one killer.

Worse still, these drugs are not necessary for most people who take them. Statin medications have been proven to cause many serious side effects, including liver failure, diabetes, cancer, and peripheral neuropathy.

RISKS ASSOCIATED WITH STATIN USE: PERIPHERAL NEUROPATHY AND BRAIN DAMAGE

It is necessary to remember that, whenever you take a prescription drug, there is a risk of side effects, including serious ones. Further, this risk multiplies every time you add another drug on top of that. Most of the patients I see are on six to twelve different prescription medications.

Under such circumstances, the odds of having a side effect of some kind are, indeed, high. Everyone is different, and it is impossible to predict how you are going to react to one prescription medication, let alone mixing half a dozen medications on a daily basis. If you are thinking that this all sounds like a recipe for potential disaster, you are quite right.

New research done in 2011 came to the following conclusion, "Long-term treatment with statins caused a clinically silent but still definite damage to peripheral nerves when the treatment lasts longer than two years."

Still not convinced? Since just 2001, there have been twelve other studies that have linked statin drug use with peripheral neuropathy. For example, a study published in *Pharmacology* in 2009 found that statin use caused damage to the brain, leading to cognitive impairment. There are more than ten studies showing the link between statin use and memory problems.

There is no doubt that this is all a little depressing, but there is some good news too. About 90 percent of the patients who were on statin drugs reported cognitive improvement after they stopped taking those medications. If you are currently taking statin drugs or considering doing so, bring these concerns up to your doctor.

CHAPTER TWO

ADDITIONAL CAUSES OF PERIPHERAL NEUROPATHY

WHAT ELSE CAN CAUSE PERIPHERAL NEUROPATHY?

Diabetes and the use of statin drugs have both been linked to peripheral neuropathy, but they are definitely not the only two factors. Another factor comes in the form of something that you probably consume each and every day. Let me explain.

There is a little known cause of peripheral neuropathy that can be found at almost every meal. This is particularly true for those who consume a diet that largely consists of processed and fast food. The culprit?

GLUTEN

Just like the link between statins and peripheral neuropathy, few people realize the link between peripheral neuropathy and gluten sensitivity. What exactly is gluten? Gluten is a protein found in wheat, and for those who have gluten-sensitivity issues, the impact of gluten on their bodies can be nothing short of profound.

In general, gluten sensitivity is used as a blanket term to describe a variety of diseases that have a common immune response to the ingestion of gluten. Here are some of the problems gluten sensitivity can cause: skin problems, such as eczema digestive problems and disorders, such as celiac disease neurological disorders, as exemplified by gluten ataxia and peripheral neuropathy

HOW MANY PEOPLE ARE AFFECTED BY GLUTEN SENSITIVITY

The exact numbers of people impacted by a sensitivity to gluten is largely unknown. The fact is that gluten hasn't received the attention it deserves in standard medical practices. However, that is slowly starting to change. Researchers are beginning to give more attention to the problem, and food manufacturers are becoming more and more aware of just how much money can be made by providing gluten-free products. Yet, despite this flurry of new attention, most people are still unaware of the connection between gluten sensitivity and peripheral neuropathy.

THREE KEY FACTS ABOUT THE NUMBER OF AMERICANS WITH GLUTEN SENSITIVITY

1. An estimated 1 in 133 people may suffer from gluten sensitivity (according to a 2004 National Institute of Health [NIH] report).
2. According to these numbers, that is almost two million people in the United States alone (NIH report).
3. Researchers estimate that twenty to thirty million Americans suffer from subclinical gluten intolerance.

14

Numbers of this magnitude tell us quite a bit. First, these statistics tell us that you more than likely know someone who has a serious issue with gluten. Secondly, with numbers this high, you may personally be in the ranks of those with gluten issues and not even know it. Third, these numbers and the fact that there is a link between peripheral neuropathy and gluten sensitivity means that millions of people are at risk.

Some experts believe no one should be consuming wheat or gluten, period.

Yet, quite alarmingly, some health experts go much further. Some experts feel that wheat is, by its very nature, inflammatory and that, to varying degrees, we are all negatively impacted by consuming it. The idea is that wheat causes a mild degree of inflammation in almost all individuals.

However, most people are able to tolerate it. Or they just attribute how they feel to other factors, such as the aches and pains of life. If it is, indeed, true that wheat and gluten protein cause inflammation in all of those who consume it, then there are serious implications for health.

I realize that wheat is difficult to avoid in the typical Western diet. After all, it is found in almost all manufactured food products. You don't have to look far to see that wheat and sugar are simply ubiquitous in processed foods. The reason for this is due to the fact that these foods are cheap and appealing to people.

These foods also negatively impact human health. Given the massive consumption of gluten and the link between peripheral neuropathy and gluten sensitivity, it is easy to see why so many people will develop peripheral neuropathy during their lifetime.

So is it possible that you are gluten intolerant? Here is a quick list of some of the most common symptoms. See if you can relate to any of these issues.

NINE OF THE WELL-KNOWN SYMPTOMS OF GLUTEN INTOLERANCE

1. abdominal pain or discomfort
2. diarrhea, including chronic diarrhea
3. constipation
4. excessive gas
5. joint pain
6. bone pain
7. muscle pain
8. bloating
9. acid reflux

There are also lesser known symptoms associated with gluten intolerance. Peripheral neuropathy and ataxia (a neurological problem that involves a lack of coordination in muscle movements) are a couple of the lesser known, and quite serious, symptoms of gluten intolerance.

As peripheral neuropathy and ataxia indicate, the problems associated with gluten intolerance can become very serious. Individuals who suspect that they have gluten issues need to take such concerns seriously.

So how big of a role could gluten intolerance be playing in the development of peripheral neuropathy? A 2006 study published in the *Journal of Neurosurgery and Psychiatry* came to some startling conclusions. In particular, this study concluded that 34 percent of those with peripheral neuropathy, whose cause could not be determined, tested positive for gluten sensitivity.

Patients are typically quite shocked to learn that something they eat every single day, something that they've consumed all of their lives, can be the root of their pain and discomfort. However, the facts are that for countless people, peripheral neuropathy can be traced back to wheat, gluten, and gluten-sensitivity issues. Addressing these issues via a change in diet can, of course, lead to amazing transformations in health, well-being, and happiness.

But gluten sensitivity clearly isn't the only culprit. There is a long list of issues that can result in peripheral neuropathy.

TWENTY-SIX OTHER CAUSES OF PERIPHERAL NEUROPATHY

– kidney disorders
– some types of cancer
– hormone imbalances
– infections and autoimmune disorders
– HIV
– herpes virus
– the bacteria that causes Lyme disease
– syphilis infection
– Guillain-Barré syndrome
– systemic lupus
– rheumatoid arthritis
– celiac disease
– some medications
– exposure to poisons
– exposure to chemicals, including industrial chemicals
– exposure to Agent Orange
– exposure to heavy metals such as mercury or lead
– chemotherapy
– vascular disorders
– circulation problems
– low levels of B vitamins
– alcoholism

– multiple sclerosis
– trauma from an injury, such as a fall, can cause nerve damage and peripheral neuropathy
– postsurgical complications can damage nerves and lead to peripheral neuropathy
– in rare circumstances, heredity

MEDICATION, POISONS, AND HEAVY-METAL EXPOSURE

People are often surprised to see the list above and learn just how many different factors can be involved in producing the damage that leads to peripheral neuropathy.

It is important to note that medication and poisons can also easily cause peripheral neuropathy. Chemotherapy not only kills cancer but also can damage the peripheral nerves.

Exposure to powerful chemicals and toxic substances, such as industrial chemicals, Agent Orange, or heavy metals (such as mercury and lead) can also cause tremendous damage. These issues can result in the damage of internal organs, such as the liver and kidneys, as well as nerve damage.

VASCULAR DISORDERS AND CIRCULATION PROBLEMS

Vascular disorders or circulation problems are also known to cause peripheral neuropathy. Poor circulation means that you have less blood flowing to your legs and feet. With these types of circulation issues comes inflammation in the blood vessels, arteriosclerosis, and other disorders. Ultimately, decreased blood flow deprives the nerves of the oxygen that they desperately need, and this leads to nerve damage and nerve-cell death.

ALCOHOLISM AND PERIPHERAL NEUROPATHY

In short, alcoholism robs the body of vital nutrients, including vitamins, such as thiamin and a handful of other essential nutrients. When key vitamins and nutrients are depleted due to alcoholism, the chances for developing peripheral neuropathy increases.

HEREDITY'S ROLE IN PERIPHERAL NEUROPATHY

In rare instances, peripheral neuropathy can be caused by heredity. The most common cause of hereditary-induced neuropathy is a condition called Charcot Marie-Tooth disease. This disease affects both the sensory and motor nerves. Charcot Marie-Tooth disease affects about one in twenty-five thousand people in the United States. The disease causes weakness—usually in the feet and lower leg muscles—and can lead to deformities.

NUTRITION, B VITAMINS, AND PERIPHERAL NEUROPATHY

A good percentage of this book will be dedicated to optimal nutrition. Striving to ensure that you are getting enough of the proper vitamins and minerals will make a difference in your health, your chances of developing peripheral neuropathy, and the severity of peripheral neuropathy.

As it turns out, a deficiency of B vitamins can play a role in the development of peripheral neuropathy. Studies have shown that individuals with low levels of B vitamins have a greater chance of developing peripheral neuropathy. So one major point of focus will be on increasing vitamin B levels through diet and supplementation.

CHAPTER THREE

DIAGNOSING NEUROPATHY

HOW IS PERIPHERAL NEUROPATHY DIAGNOSED?

The steps to diagnosing any disease or condition can be quite involved. Many factors and elements must be taken into consideration to ensure an accurate diagnosis. This is why it is essential for professionals to obtain a proper medical history. Additionally, performing a physical examination is essential.

We always inform our new patients that they should be ready to discuss all of their symptoms in detail during their initial appointment. This process entails describing their symptoms, when they experience these symptoms, how long symptoms last, and the amount of discomfort or pain. The more specific that a patient is regarding his or her symptoms—such as burning, numbness, or tingling—the easier it will be for a doctor to understand your peripheral neuropathy.

Part of the diagnostic process is to ask a range of general health questions that may seem unrelated. But these questions are vital nonetheless.

It is our goal to understand if you are suffering from any other conditions and what kinds of medications you are on. Encouraging a patient to outline his or her family history is also significant, as some neuropathies can be inherited.

The initial examination includes evaluating the sensory nerves in the extremities. This involves a doctor testing your ability to feel different types of stimuli, for example, being able to perceive hot and cold on your feet or hands. At this stage, a doctor should also check your ability to feel sharp and light touches. Also, your doctor will check your sense of balance.

Your response to these different tests will indicate which nerves are damaged and how severe the damage is. In addition to these physical tests, it is possible that your doctor might also order blood work to look for underlying causes of neuropathy.

Between the physical exam and medical history, a doctor is usually able to get a good idea of whether or not the patient has peripheral neuropathy. Blood work can be quite valuable, as it helps to identify possible causes for the peripheral neuropathy.

NEUROLOGISTS

Sometimes patients will be referred to a neurologist. Neurologists are medical doctors who specialize in the nervous system. Neurologists perform two different kinds of nerve tests. The first is an NCV (nerve-conduction velocity test), and the second is an EMG (electromyogram test). The NCV measures the rate that the nerve impulse travels and is quite useful, as it can detect nerve damage. The EMG tests muscles' response to a nerve being stimulated and can detect a neuromuscular problem.

WHAT ARE THE COMPLICATIONS WITH PERIPHERAL NEUROPATHY?

Peripheral neuropathy patients face many challenges. At the top of the list is losing feeling in their feet. This symptom is reported a great deal and can have a range of significant implications.

Not being able to feel your feet also means that you are not able to sense the ground as you are walking. This, of course, means that you will not have full balance and coordination. Most activities involving mobility, such as walking, become problematic. For patients who can't feel their feet, some form of assistance is generally required, whether it means opting for a cane, a walker, or a wheelchair.

A REDUCTION IN MOBILITY AND QUALITY OF LIFE

This reduction in mobility will usually be linked to other health issues, such as reduced cardiovascular fitness. Problems with mobility also usually mean spending less time outdoors. This quickly translates to a decrease in vitamin D levels due to less sun exposure. Peripheral neuropathy patients will typically experience reduced cardiovascular health and accompanying weight gain.

A decrease in mobility is far more complicated and serious of an issue than simply needing a cane, walker, or even a wheelchair. The truth is that a loss of mobility means a decrease in both quality of life and overall health. It can potentially even impact longevity.

The loss of sensation in the feet and legs can affect a person's quality of life and mobility in some unexpected ways. For example, patients often lose their ability to drive a car. Since patients are unable to distinguish the gas pedal from the brake, driving a car becomes hazardous. In fact, peripheral neuropathy often plays a role in the elderly losing their driver's licenses. With the loss of their license, they also lose a good deal of freedom and independence.

All of these factors I've outlined point to why peripheral neuropathy is such a significant problem and should be treated immediately and with the utmost seriousness. Yet there is still one more problem to add to the mix, and it comes in the form of amputations.

AN ELEVATED RISK FOR AMPUTATION

Unfortunately, there is a link between amputations and peripheral neuropathy. Once one loses sensation in the bottom of the foot, the odds of infection increase.

Here's the reason: if you have less circulation to an area of your body, there is a reduced ability for the body to fight infection. For example, people with numb feet often step on something sharp, like glass, and don't feel it. This can develop into an infection and progress to gangrene. The final result of this process can be amputation. This surgery, in turn, means even less mobility and a further worsening of the problems outlined above, such as weight gain, decreased cardiovascular health, and an overall decrease in fitness and quality of life.

Eighty-six thousand amputations occur every single year, mostly associated to peripheral neuropathy and peripheral vascular disease.

Let's put this into context. If there were eighty-six thousand amputations as a result of a war every year, we would definitely be hearing about that war. Eighty-six thousand is a remarkably high number. It means that over a ten-year period, almost a million people will have had amputations as a result of peripheral neuropathy or peripheral vascular disease.

CHAPTER FOUR

DIABETIC NEUROPATHY

Microvascular disease is the main causes of diabetic neuropathy.

For diabetics, the feet are a real issue, as most develop neuropathy in their feet. The tiny little nerves and blood vessels are of concern. These blood vessels are called micro-capillaries, and the nerves and the microcirculation are closely related and intertwined. Blood vessels depend on normal nerve function, and nerves depend on adequate blood flow.

Proper blood flow is essential for good health. With diabetics, the biggest challenge is decreased blood flow. Diabetics develop peripheral vascular disease, which results in diminished blood flow.

This diminished blood flow first shows up in the extremities because circulation is easier to disrupt in the limbs than in the rest of the body. In part, this is due to the fact that the feet are so far away from the heart. When micro–blood vessels are damaged, the nerves do not get enough nutrients and oxygen. Severe nerve damage can result.

There is also a condition called neuro-ischemia that can develop. This essentially means that nerves are not getting enough oxygen. The blood vessels actually constrict in a process called vasoconstriction. As a result, not enough blood reaches the nerve endings to keep them healthy.

A second major factor impacting diabetics is that they have the challenge of high blood-glucose levels, which are significant in some key ways. The first is that high blood-glucose levels cause an increase in the amount of free radicals. These free radicals cause cell damage and premature aging. Secondly, high blood sugar depletes the cells of glutathione.

THE VITAL IMPORTANCE OF GLUTATHIONE

Glutathione neutralizes free radicals in the body. Your cells make glutathione, and it is the most powerful antioxidant in your body.

This essential antioxidant helps decrease inflammation in the body and serves to regulate nitric oxide. Healthy nitric oxide levels are the key to having good blood flow.

High glucose levels in the bloodstream can cause a variety of problems. They can affect the body's ability to regulate glutathione and antioxidant levels. The body also starts to have trouble regulating the nitric-oxide cycle, which is critical for life and health of the nerves.

CHAPTER FIVE

THE DIFFERENT FACES OF PERIPHERAL NEUROPATHY

When patients come into my office with a diagnosis of neuropathy, their condition may be in any one of a variety of stages. If they are experiencing just slight numbness or tingling in the toes or the balls of their feet, they are likely in the earliest stage. At this stage, it feels like more of a nuisance than anything. Patients don't realize it's an early warning sign of a potentially serious condition.

During the earliest stages of the condition, peripheral neuropathy does not hamper an individual's life; it's not affecting their balance, and it's not having an impact on their ability to do things they enjoy. This means that their mobility has not yet been impaired. As a result, patients usually don't pursue diagnosis and treatment options early on. Many feel that the numbness or tingling that they feel is just a slight annoyance, and they try to ignore it. Of course, this is unfortunate. When it comes to peripheral neuropathy, the sooner diagnosis and treatment is pursued, the better.

As time goes on, those symptoms typically worsen in intensity, location, and duration. If a patient were just suffering from slight numbness, the peripheral neuropathy would progress to the point where it causes severe numbness in the ball of the foot and in the toes. Or it can start to encompass the entire bottom or top of the feet. It is this stark progression that usually gets a person's attention.

Burning sensations are the number-one symptom that drives sufferers of peripheral neuropathy to finally seek out medical attention. When patients have severe enough burning in their feet, or what many refer to as "hot feet," they usually turn to their doctor to find out exactly what is going on.

It will generally start in the front of the feet, in the toes and the ball. Next it progresses up to the entire foot. Eventually peripheral neuropathy will start going across the ankle and up the leg. When this happens, the balance issues become noticeable.

Why does peripheral neuropathy cause a lack of balance? This is due to the fact that the nerves responsible for controlling balance, proprioceptive nerves, become damaged. The proprioceptive nerves are responsible for telling the brain the position of the foot, your ankle, your toes, and your knee. When these critical nerves are damaged, coordination is affected, and a person's gait changes. Patients experience a noticeable difference in how they walk and move.

This loss of normal balanced movement is what causes people to become what some refer to as "wall walkers." Patients frequently tell me that, when they walk down the hall, they have no choice but to put their hands on the wall to keep their balance. Additionally, their spouses, friends, and relatives will often report that they see changes in the way they walk, such as a wobbling that one would typically associate with falling.

All of these symptoms lead us to the issue of falling and all the concerns that come with it.

As peripheral neuropathy progresses to this point, the risk of falling is great. Falling down, of course, means the potential for significant injury. Since the majority of peripheral neuropathy sufferers are elderly, fractures due to falls can take a long time to heal and can lead to a variety of health complications.

Patients enter our office in various stages of peripheral neuropathy. In order to best address their specific needs, we assess what stage they are in. For example, there is the initial stage, where the nerve damage is minimal. Patients are just having slight symptoms.

When I see a patient with numbness, tingling, and burning sensations in their feet or their toes, I describe it as "initial-stage peripheral neuropathy." If they have lots of numbness, where it feels like they have a piece of leather on the bottom of their feet or it feels like something's rolled up in their sock, this is severe peripheral neuropathy. These patients can barely feel the ground. This factor begins to limit their ability to walk safely or, for that matter, drive a car.

The issue of driving and peripheral neuropathy is one that many people overlook for a range of reasons, but it is actually quite significant for the safety of everyone on the road.

For example, I once had a patient who told me that he drove by sound— the sound of the engine, that is. He could tell by the idle sound and the rev of the engine just how much pressure he had on the gas pedal. Comforting, right? One day he pulled into a restaurant, and he thought he hit the brake; instead he hit the gas and ran right into the side of the restaurant. This event finally motivated him to seek some help for his problem.

Typically, peripheral neuropathy starts in the front of the feet, the toes, or the ball of the foot, and it slowly works into the entire foot and then up the leg. The exact symptoms are different for everybody. Some patients strictly have numbness, with no associated pain. In these patients, peripheral neuropathy starts with numbness and develops into balance issues.

For other patients, the progression of peripheral neuropathy differs. It may begin with muscle cramping in the feet and/or calves. Adding yet another layer of complexity is the fact that sometimes the progression of peripheral neuropathy is strictly related to pain.

These patients experience a burning sensation in their feet. Often they cannot even wear shoes due to this intense burning sensation. In order to cope with this pain, these patients usually wear a sandal-style shoe. They usually have a severe problem at night, as they have no choice but to sleep with their legs outside the covers because their feet get so hot. In fact, I've had patients tell me that they'll put a fan at the end of the bed to cool their feet. Some patients get up in the middle of night and put their feet into buckets of ice; that's how bad the pain is.

CHAPTER SIX

COMMON MEDICATIONS FOR PERIPHERAL NEUROPATHY

As we discussed earlier in this book, all medications have side effects. These side effects can range from mild to severe and even be life threatening. It is no coincidence that the medication commercials you see on television are one-part commercial and two-part legal disclaimer that outlines the "rare but possible" occasions in which severe side effects may occur. If the side effects weren't so serious, it would be the stuff of good comic fodder. But the side effects of these drugs are potentially very serious.

It will come as no surprise that there are many drugs used to treat peripheral neuropathy. Most of the patients who come into my office are taking at least a few different drugs. By the time I see most patients, they have typically have gone through the standard of care. For painful peripheral neuropathy, the general routine is to see doctors who prescribe a few different medications.

GABAPENTIN/NEURONTIN

The most popular medication for peripheral neuropathy is called gabapentin; its brand name is Neurontin. It is important to note that this medication is actually FDA cleared for seizure disorders. Doctors prescribe Neurontin for peripheral neuropathy because it distracts the patient from thinking about his or her feet. It doesn't fix the problem. It slows your brain down so you don't get the feedback of pain—intense burning or electrical shock sensations—as these feelings are sent from the feet to the brain.

It is quite important to point out that Neurontin is *not* FDA approved to treat peripheral neuropathy. However, this is the most popularly prescribed drug for managing the pain of peripheral neuropathy. **Remember that no drug can currently *cure* peripheral neuropathy.**

In fact, Pfizer, the company that makes Neurontin, actually had to settle two different lawsuits for a total of half a billion dollars. They were sued because the government discovered that Pfizer was marketing drugs for the express purpose of treating peripheral neuropathy. Pfizer was violating the law because Neurontin was being promoted to doctors as a treatment for neuropathy. As I explained above, Neurontin has only been approved for treating seizure disorders.

Yet, in what can only be called an amazing twist, Neurontin, to this day, still remains the most popularly prescribed drug for peripheral neuropathy. Patients who are on Neurontin for their peripheral neuropathy, even though it is not FDA approved, come to us every day.

LYRICA, AMITRIPTYLINE, AND PERIPHERAL NEUROPATHY

The second medication that is prescribed for neuropathy is called Lyrica. Like Neurontin, Lyrica is also an antiseizure medication. There is one significant difference, however, in that Lyrica is approved by the FDA to treat peripheral neuropathy. A third drug commonly prescribed for peripheral neuropathy is an antidepressant called Amitriptyline.

Peripheral neuropathy is a degenerative condition, meaning it gets worse with time. As it gets worse, the symptoms tend to intensify. So when a patient actually experiences severe pain from peripheral neuropathy, the medications discussed above tend to do very little to relieve symptoms and pain. The standard antiseizure medications, such as Neurontin and Lyrica, or the antidepressants, such as Amitriptyline, have no real impact. These patients instead gravitate toward opting for pain management, which comes with its own problems.

The move toward the pain-management spectrum is quite problematic, as it means that peripheral neuropathy patients are given powerful and potentially highly addictive drugs. These drugs include Vicodin, Norco, or OxyContin. Unfortunately, the typical treatment for people with severe peripheral neuropathy is to prescribe narcotics.

NARCOTICS DO NOT ADDRESS THE CAUSE OF PERIPHERAL NEUROPATHY

Drugs, such as Vicodin and OxyContin, do not address peripheral neuropathy. Instead, these drugs only serve to offer temporary relief of symptoms. What choices do patients in need of help have?

Most suffering from peripheral neuropathy either live with pain and potentially decreased mobility, diminished overall health, and weight gain or opt for narcotics and get some temporary relief from their pain. Yet it is important to note that the narcotic route for pain relief is one with no end in sight. In short, patients will be taking pain medication for the rest of their lives. Even more troubling, patients can expect to increase their dosage as symptoms worsen, which they invariably almost always will.

Then there is the issue of side effects and combining multiple drugs. Antiseizure drugs come with a big list of side effects. Adding drugs, such as Vicodin, into the mix further complicates an already complex situation.

PHARMACEUTICAL PAIN RELIEF DRUGS COME WITH SIDE EFFECTS

I see a lot of serious side effects when it comes to peripheral neuropathy patients who are taking prescription pain killers, and it's not pretty. The most common side effects that I witness are dizziness, fatigue, weight gain, drowsiness, and swelling in the legs and ankles. Now, keep in mind that these side effects are usually being seen in elderly patients who often already have other medical conditions.

It is also important to note that, when I say drowsiness, I mean extreme drowsiness, as if patients are taking drugs for recreation. In short, these patients are not functioning at a normal level cognitively. These patients have slower speech patterns and movements and are not, for all practical purposes, themselves.

Spouses of patients always tell me that their loved one used to be energetic but that the drugs sapped the life right out of them. The reality is that those taking these drugs become mostly sedentary. They largely abandon the things that they once enjoyed. The bottom line is that the side effects of these drugs are more than just serious; sometimes they are worse than the disease being treated with these drugs.

MOOD SWINGS, SUICIDAL THOUGHTS, AND ACTS LINKED TO PERIPHERAL NEUROPATHY DRUGS

Mood swings are a very common side effect from use of peripheral-neuropathy drugs. Difficulty concentrating and hostility are common.

Alarmingly, there is a link between suicidal acts and violent deaths as well. In 2009, the FDA issued a warning of increased risk of depression and suicidal thoughts and behaviors in patients taking Gabapentin.

Lyrica has numerous side effects, the most common being dizziness, drowsiness, fatigue, blurred vision, increased appetite, confusion, decreased libido, erectile dysfunction, and worse memory, coordination, and balance.

As we discussed, Amitriptyline is an antidepressant often prescribed to patients with peripheral neuropathy. The most common side effects associated with Amitriptyline are weight gain, muscle stiffness, nausea, nervousness, constipation, dizziness, decreased libido, and pain or numbness in the feet or hands.

Amitriptyline causes pain and numbness in the hands? Isn't that exactly what we are trying to get rid of in the first place? Amitriptyline is given for peripheral neuropathy, but the drug has side effects that are identical to the condition itself.

CHAPTER SEVEN

STANDARD MEDICAL TREATMENT

When a patient is experiencing symptoms of peripheral neuropathy, he or she usually seeks the help of a physician. But patients usually wait until their symptoms are more advanced before making the trip. Depending on the physician and based on the symptoms and history of the patient, the doctor will give the patient prescriptions for these medications. However, if the physician is not comfortable managing peripheral neuropathy, the patient will be referred to a neurologist, where he or she will undergo diagnostic testing.

HOW DOES A NEUROLOGIST HELP?

There are two tests that neurologists typically perform when addressing peripheral neuropathy. One is a nerve-conduction test, and the other is called an electromyogram. These tests help document the level of nerve damage, and then based on that information, a neurologist will prescribe pain medication or tell the patient there are no options but to live with the numbness.

If you are thinking that this doesn't seem like a lot of options, well you are, of course, correct. **Doctors typically tell patients with peripheral neuropathy that there's nothing that can be done and that it will get worse.** This is the current standard care for treating peripheral neuropathy.

Option A is to manage the pain with medication. If there is no pain but only numbness, then option B is to live with it and provide a cane or walker when balance starts to fail.

Finally, in cases where infections arise from ulcerations in the feet, wound care is performed. If necessary, toes, feet, and lower limbs are amputated. This isn't a pretty picture, but it is an accurate assessment of the state of standard-care treatment for peripheral neuropathy.

CHAPTER EIGHT

FOUR CRITICAL MISTAKES TO AVOID WHEN CHOOSING AN ALTERNATIVE PROVIDER

ALTERNATIVE HEALTH CARE IS INCREASINGLY POPULAR

Nearly 40 percent of adults already use alternative treatments to resolve health problems, and the numbers are growing. The reason being that people aren't satisfied with the standard medical approach of just treating symptoms and not fixing the cause. Patients are achieving impressive results in treating a range of conditions and illnesses with alternative health care.

Alternative care can be used alone or in combination with other medications and treatments. Of all the alternative health-care providers, chiropractors are the most popular providers of complementary and alternative treatments.

Eighty percent of medical doctors say alternative medicine is useful for pain management but that their busy practices make it difficult to stay on top of the latest alternative treatments and therapies. Many physicians are broadening their referral base to include holistic practitioners in treating peripheral neuropathy, and they are helping patients achieve impressive results in the process.

I must assume that if you're reading this book, you are not satisfied with just taking medicine to cover up your symptoms. Finding the right alternative practitioner for your peripheral neuropathy can truly make all the difference in the world. As we have discussed, the impact that peripheral neuropathy can make on your quality of life and well-being can be profound. Selecting the right health-care professional to help you address your peripheral neuropathy is of great importance.

You should select an experienced health-care provider who focuses most, if not *all*, of his or her practice time on helping peripheral-neuropathy patients. If you had cancer, you wouldn't go to a doctor who dabbles in treating cancer on a part-time basis. You should treat your peripheral neuropathy in the same way. You need a practitioner who is an expert and dedicates 100 percent of his or her time to helping patients with neuropathy. It is important to note that most chiropractors and physicians do not focus on peripheral neuropathy.

Many factors contribute to peripheral neuropathy and its severity, and that means a comprehensive approach is the best option. The most effective providers use a combination of safe and effective therapies and treatments to address causes and symptoms of peripheral neuropathy.

With this being said, I meet countless patients who have gone to alternative practitioners but had zero results from their care. Here are the most common mistakes people make with alternative providers.

FOUR CRITICAL MISTAKES WHEN CHOOSING AN ALTERNATIVE TREATMENT FOR NEUROPATHY

Knowing these four mistakes will help you to avoid them and select the right treatment. This will save you much aggravation—not to mention time and money.

MISTAKE ONE: TREATMENT DOESN'T INCREASE BLOOD FLOW TO MICRO-BLOOD VESSELS (CAPILLARIES) IN THE FEET AND LEGS

One of the causes of neuropathy and the reason it gets worse is because the tiny blood vessels (capillaries) in the feet and legs are damaged. These blood vessels wrap around the nerves and are the nerve's life source. The blood flow brings oxygen and nutrients to the nerve. If you cut the blood flow off to the nerve, it will begin to die.

Decreased blood flow is the main cause for neuropathy and the primary reason it gets worse with time.

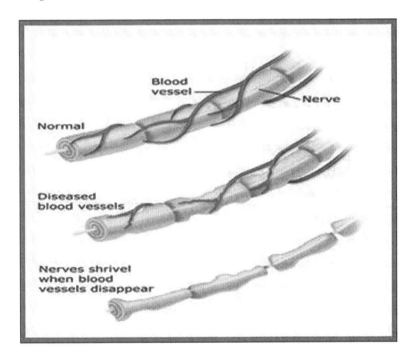

If you want any chance of reducing or ending your pain or numbness, you must select a treatment protocol that will increase the blood flow to your legs and feet.

41

The best technology to increase blood flow to the feet is LED light therapy. LED light therapy is FDA cleared to increase circulation and decrease pain. There have been over two thousand studies showing the benefits of light therapy. I think it's interesting to mention that NASA has done extensive research on this treatment technology. If you are a research hound like me, you can take a look at NASA's research on LED therapy at http://www.msfc.nasa.gov.

The way LED light therapy works is very interesting. It uses a specific wavelength of red (650 nm) and infrared (880 nm) light. These wavelengths cause damaged blood vessels to dilate, which causes more blood to get to the nerves. What this means is that now your nerves have a fighting chance, because they will get more nutrition and oxygen from the increased blood flow. Also, it causes angiogenesis. This means the LED light stimulates your body to grow more blood vessels. This increases the blood flow to your nerves, even when you're not getting treatment.

* *

Don't make the mistake of going to a practitioner who uses a handheld laser to treat neuropathy. Handheld lasers are designed for deep treatment of joints and muscles. These lasers do a great job for treating parts of the body where pain is focused, like a shoulder or elbow. With peripheral neuropathy, the problem is over a large area of the foot, hands, or legs. It's difficult to deliver an even dosage of light therapy to an entire foot or leg with a handheld laser. Also, it is easy to aggravate neuropathy if you are not precise with the dosage and power of the light source.

MISTAKE TWO: TREATMENT DOESN'T STIMULATE DAMAGED NERVES

An alternative provider should be able provide safe pain relief without risky prescription drugs.

When the sensory nerves in your feet or legs are damaged, they atrophy (shrink). This is similar to what happens to your muscles after you get a cast removed from your leg or arm. Your muscles atrophy; they get smaller. This process will cause pain and/or numbness.

Typically, the standard of care for neuropathy pain is prescription medications to mask the symptoms. Instead of prescription drugs, an alternative provider should use advanced, safe, and painless electrical-stimulation treatment.

There are a lot of different electrical-stimulation devices on the market. It's important to know that most of them are very low tech and don't have good results. I have had patients go out and purchase a standard two to three hundred–dollar electrical-stimulation unit for home use. It didn't work and was a waste of money.

This isn't what I'm talking about.

What I'm referring to is the latest in German technology, a computer-driven treatment that delivers a patented frequency technology to your damaged nerves. This technology exercises your nerves (neuromuscular reeducation). This is critical when you're trying to rehabilitate damaged nerves. You have to get your nerves working again electrically.

MISTAKE THREE: YOUR DOCTOR DOESN'T ADDRESS NUTRITION

There are specific nutritional protocols that must be followed for good results. In fact, the foods you are eating could cause your neuropathy to worsen. Your doctor must provide a comprehensive nutritional and supplement program for you. Without it, you may not get any results—or minimal results at best.

Your doctor should have the specialized knowledge to identify the foods you may be eating that can contribute to your neuropathy and make it worse.

Some foods promote inflammation of the nerves and decrease peripheral circulation at the same time. Some foods can cause an autoimmune reaction within neuropathy sufferers.

There are specialized nutritional supplements that help reduce inflammation and increase peripheral circulation. These supplements help increase your glutathione leves. This is critical to getting optimal results with a comprehensive neuropathy treatment program.

Glutathione is the largest antioxidant in the body and is nothing short of essential. Each cell of your body produces glutathione. Chronic inflammatory conditions reduce the level of glutathione in the body. This, in turn, becomes quite problematic.

Lower glutathione levels lead to a free-radical buildup in the body. In turn, this causes more damage. Patients will suffer from more cellular and **nerve damage,** as well as more damage to the arteries and the capillaries, inhibiting circulation, and so on. The goal should be to slow down or stop this process to see real and lasting improvement.

The world at large works to deplete glutathione levels, as everything from stress to pollution take a toll. Evidence also shows that our glutathione levels decrease dramatically with age and chronic health problems.

Finding out what you can do to increase your glutathione levels is essential in protecting your health. Low glutathione levels are associated with a range of diseases and conditions, but the good news is that there are steps you can take to keep your glutathione levels high.

FOUR WAYS TO INCREASE YOUR GLUTATHIONE LEVELS

1. Eat more garlic, onions, and cruciferous vegetables, like broccoli, kale, cabbage, and cauliflower.
2. Increase the amount of exercise you do daily.
3. Supplement with acetyl-glutathione. This is the only form of glutathione that your body can absorb. Read the glutathione-supplement facts carefully. It must be in the form of acetyl-glutathione, or your body can't absorb it.
4. Supplement with the building blocks of glutathione, such as alpha lipoic acid, acetylcysteine, glutamine, and selenium.

ALPHA LIPOIC ACID

Alpha lipoic acid, or ALA, is absolutely essential for the production of glutathione. ALA is very beneficial for treating diabetic peripheral neuropathy. If you are a diabetic, you will certainly want to take this supplement as part of your approach toward improving your health and addressing your peripheral neuropathy.

N-ACETYLCYSTEINE

Another building block of glutathione comes in the form of N-acetylcysteine. Some research indicates that N-acetylcysteine may boost the immune system as well.

L-GLUTAMINE

A third glutathione-building supplement is L-glutamine. L-glutamine is an amino acid frequently used in the body-building world, as it can improve performance. Additionally, L-glutamine may also play a role in the treatment of chronic inflammation diseases, such as ulcerative colitis. Evidence indicates that L-glutamine may speed up recovery from injury.

SELENIUM

Why is selenium important? As it turns out, selenium performs a pretty nifty trick in that it can help your body not only produce more glutathione but also recycle existing glutathione.

VITAMIN B

Finally, stable vitamin B-1 and B-12 levels are essential for healthy nerves. Benfotiamine is a special form of vitamin B1 and been shown to be effective in treating some painful nerve conditions.

The best providers for treating peripheral neuropathic pain are those who treat the whole body rather than just focusing on specific pain symptoms. A skilled practitioner will carefully evaluate the patient and create a treatment plan to address the underlying conditions that may be causing neuropathic symptoms. Be sure to select a professional who spends a substantial amount of time evaluating you and your condition.

For example, when a new peripheral-neuropathy patient comes to see me, I am sure to conduct a very thorough analysis of his or her history and current conditions. I spend time getting to know my patient and his or her lifestyle and various routines. Successful holistic treatments are often geared toward helping patients make dietary changes, manage blood sugar, take appropriate supplements, and perform selected exercises.

Finally, it's important that your primary physician keeps an eye on the medications you take during alternative treatment. Many times, a patient's medications need to be decreased or eliminated after he or she starts feeling better as a result of the comprehensive alternative-care program—especially if the program includes diet modifications.

Ultimately, you want to find a healthcare provider with a proven track record of success.

CHAPTER NINE

THE STRAW PROTOCOL

There is a very large and growing demand for alternative-therapy providers in the United States, especially a demand for alternative care for neuropathy sufferers.

It is important to note that we have helped over three thousand patients in the last three years making us the largest alternative provider of peripheral-neuropathy treatment in California and quite possibly the whole United States. In my Southern California offices alone, we have fifteen doctors dedicating 100 percent of their time to helping people find the relief they have been seeking for so long. I don't say this to impress you but to impress upon you that you aren't alone—that thousands of patients have come before you seeking relief.

If a physician's only tool to treat peripheral neuropathy results in debilitating pain with no promise of a better future, then it's time to take a look at other options. Fortunately, there is another option in the form of a four-part regimen that has shown considerable promise where medication fails. This is called the **Straw Protocol**.

The Straw Protocol is a comprehensive, noninvasive treatment program designed to help patients who suffer with neuropathy. Treating nerve pain with only medication can lead to dependency and side effects that cause more harm than good.

The first step of the Straw Protocol is drug-free pain relief and nerve rehabilitation. We use a specific computerized treatment device called Hakomed. It delivers a patented frequency technology to damaged nerves. This is not only a safe approach for relief from nerve pain, but the technology also helps to rehabilitate the damaged-nerve pain.

Hakomed nerve stimulation is an effective way to address damaged nerves. This treatment uses computer-modulated electronic signals to decrease nerve pain and increase your ability to feel your feet. This treatment process helps improve the connection between the nerves in your feet and your brain. Specifically, there are specialized nerves called proprioceptive nerves in your feet, ankles, and knees. These nerves are responsible for telling your brain where your feet are. When treatment begins to work, balance begins to improve.

The second step in the Straw Protocol is to increase circulation with LED light therapy. The Straw Protocol utilizes a LED light–therapy system that is designed specifically for the feet and hands. This is a critical treatment that works to help the body get more blood to the feet and/or hands. Infrared light has been found to stimulate nitric-oxide release and cause local vasodilation, which improves circulation and helps to heal the damaged nerves.

Microcirculation involves the circulation of the smallest blood vessels and capillaries in the body. By promoting this type of circulation, low-level light therapy can assist the surrounding never fibers. As the light starts to stimulate the area, it causes more blood flow, which brings more oxygen and nutrients. This is essential to nerve health, and over time, this process causes the formation of new micro–blood vessels in the area. This helps to increase blood flow long after treatment has been completed. Simply stated, pharmaceutical pain drugs can't achieve these kinds of results.

FIVE ESSENTIAL WAYS THAT LIGHT THERAPY HAS BEEN SHOWN TO BOOST HEALTH

1. Reduces pain
2. Improves circulation
3. Accelerates healing
4. Increases production of DNA and collagen
5. Improves immune function

The facts are that low-level light therapy is a viable alternative to pain medications for the treatment of peripheral neuropathy. This therapy is highly effective and is used by well-informed medical doctors, osteopaths, and chiropractors as an alternative to pain medications. When used as part of a comprehensive treatment plan, low-level light therapy improves blood flow, helps to restore sensation, and reduces pain for patients with diabetic peripheral neuropathy.

Step three is vibration therapy. What makes vibration therapy so attractive is that it has been shown to increase circulation to the feet and stimulate the nerves that help with balance.

Vibration therapy works to activate the same nerves that control balance, which makes this therapy invaluable. Further adding benefit to vibration therapy is the fact that it stimulates local circulation by increasing blood flow. Again, boosting blood flow is essential for effectively addressing peripheral neuropathy.

Food choices and specific supplementation play a very important role in a comprehensive neuropathy-treatment program. The right dietary choices combined with select supplementation can make a massive difference in how your body responds to your peripheral neuropathy.

At the heart of the Straw Protocol is changing what patients eat, their approach to food, and their approach to supplementation. Patients with peripheral neuropathy have chronic inflammation in the nerves, their blood vessels, and their micro-capillaries. As a result, switching to a low-inflammation diet is vital. Let's take a look at the foundation of a low-inflammation diet.

THE TEN CORE ELEMENTS OF A LOW-INFLAMMATION DIET

1. Low in DNA-damaging sugar
2. As few processed foods as possible
3. Low in grains, such as wheat, which can trigger inflammation
4. Eliminate processed fats and trans fats
5. Eliminate harmful artificial sweeteners
6. Eliminate harmful additives found in processed foods, such as dyes and chemicals
7. Increase water intake and opt for purified water if possible
8. Eat foods that decrease inflammation in the body
9. Eat foods that are rich in vitamins, minerals, and antioxidants
10. Eat healthy whole foods with a focus on vegetables of many different colors, nuts, seeds, and low-fat proteins or protein choices that are high in omega-3 fatty acids, such as sardines, wild Alaskan salmon, and walnuts

By adopting these ten, low-inflammation diet options, patients will experience many positive outcomes. Following a low-inflammation diet may help improve circulation, increase overall energy levels, decrease depression levels, help rid the body of toxins, and, of course, lower levels of inflammation.

It is important to note that most people have been living with some degree of inflammation. This is a result of their dietary and lifestyle choices. This has been going on for so long that they don't even realize inflammation is the key underlying cause of their chronic poor health. The daily aches and random pains that so many of us feel are actually a byproduct of our diets.

A diet that causes inflammation is one that is constantly working *against* the body. The right food choices will help the body rebuild. That is exactly why a low-inflammation diet is of such great importance in the Straw Protocol.

CONTROLLING AND REDUCING INFLAMMATION OPENS UP NEW HEALTH OPTIONS

Once a patient feels better, thanks to different dietary choices, it is possible for the body to begin playing a more dynamic role in healing. Next it becomes possible to exercise. This step begins moving the entire process in a new and exciting direction. In time, a patient is able to walk a mile instead of a block. This builds up stamina and improves circulation, which, of course, aids in addressing peripheral neuropathy.

Low-level light therapy, Hakomed nerve stimulation, vibration therapy, and our eating plan work together to improve patients' quality of life by decreasing pain and increasing their ability to remain active. This is done with almost no risk of harmful side effects.

Patients increase circulation, decrease pain, and improve their balance. This leads to a potentially better and longer life. The Straw Protocol helps to return people whose lives have been negatively impacted by peripheral neuropathy to being active and living the life they enjoy.

OUR APPROACH

Our approach and mission are geared toward one thing and one thing only: results. Let's take a look at how our methodology yields consistent results for our patients.

1. We provide **drug-free holistic natural treatments to lessen nerve damage, decrease pain, regain balance, and help patients enjoy more independence and an active lifestyle.**
2. Our mission is to dramatically improve the health of people living with peripheral neuropathy. As a result, **our entire focus is on treating individuals suffering with peripheral neuropathy.**
3. We lead the way in providing **innovative therapies and highly targeted customized care.**
4. We're committed to helping seniors achieve pain relief and improved health by providing powerful treatments, helpful information, and personalized support.
5. **We recognize that the best treatments may vary from person to person,** so we work closely with our patients to promote health and wellness, provide patient education, and offer customized treatments for unique peripheral-neuropathy symptoms.
6. When it comes to effectively treating peripheral neuropathy, information is everything. Not only do we carefully listen to your feedback, but you can also trust us to stay informed on the latest and most effective strategies and therapies for treating peripheral neuropathy. This protocol allows us to deliver **optimal outcomes for each individual.**

7. Over the course of our ten-week program, we see our patients as many as thirty times. We provide individualized education and coaching to help our patients take a more active role in managing their health and neuropathy.

8. **During this ten-week program, we utilize a variety of treatments and therapies to put our patients on the road to recovery and wellness.** These treatments and therapies include everything from low-level light therapy, dietary counseling, and supplementation to targeted exercises, vibration treatments, and electrotherapeutic stimulation.

EXPECT TREATMENT THAT WORKS!

A critical and unique part of our treatment plan involves dietary-supplement interventions that help patients lower their blood-sugar levels, maintain a healthier weight, and decrease pain. With a problematic condition like peripheral neuropathy, it is critical to provide patients with the opportunity to improve their health and quality of life, and that is exactly what we achieve time and time again for our patients. This often means looking beyond the scope of traditional medicine. Our view is that, in the end, what matters are results, not dogma or following the status quo. Most medical physicians agree that giving patients more choices, responsibilities, and control in their own treatment will improve the level of care.

CHAPTER TEN

THE OPTIMAL-HEALTH EATING PLAN

THE SENSIBLE AND HEALTHY WAY TO EAT FOR A LIFETIME OF OPTIMAL HEALTH AND HEALING

Most individuals with peripheral neuropathy require an advanced diet to restore health and healing to their bodies. I call this program The Optimal-Health Eating Plan. We have found that the patients that get the best results in my offices are the ones that follow this diet closely. This way of eating is critical for long term health not just during their healing phase of care. Long after patients finish their care plans we find the diet helps prevent neuropathy symptoms from returning.

Please note that I am realistic and know that most people don't follow this eating plan one hundred percent of the time. Most patients that follow this diet seventy to eighty percent of the time get outstanding results.

WHAT MAKES THIS EATING PLAN SO POWERFUL AND WORTHWHILE?

This diet works by utilizing two principals: increasing good fats and removing sugar and everything that turns to sugar (grains). These principles allow this diet to benefit your body in a way that other plans are simply not capable of doing.

THREE FUNCTIONS OF THE OPTIMAL-HEALTH EATING PLAN

Following this diet accomplishes three objectives: removing toxins, regulating hormone function, and controlling inflammation, which in turn promote healing. In my view, inflammation is the major underlying cause of most new millennium diseases.

USING FOOD TO LOWER INFLAMMATION AND BOOST HEALTH

It is almost impossible to be truly healthy or feel well if you are eating foods that trigger inflammation. Even those who are in perfect health will feel the impact of following a diet that triggers inflammation. The aches and pains that many people feel throughout the day and believe are a normal part of existence are, in fact, directly related to diet.

We have touched on the importance of opting for a low-inflammation diet. The bottom line is that anyone can benefit from such a diet, and those with peripheral neuropathy stand to benefit greatly. Let's briefly recap the most important aspects of a low-inflammation diet.

A LOW-INFLAMMATION DIET IS IN YOUR BEST INTEREST

As you can see, the core components of a low-inflammation diet differ considerably from the diet that most people in the Western world currently consume. Yet the bottom line is that a low-inflammation diet is one that is packed with good stuff and largely missing the bad stuff. As a result, you can be quite sure that your body will respond in a positive fashion.

A low-inflammation diet is one that doesn't just help address the pains and causes of peripheral neuropathy but can also help people lose weight, boost immunity, and may even help address other existing medical conditions, such as wounds that are slow or refuse to heal. Being in constant inflammation is simply horrible for the body, as it keeps your neuropathy from healing. This situation, of course, contributes to the worsening symptoms of peripheral neuropathy.

What you eat matters. Under no circumstances should you allow anyone to convince you that what you eat doesn't matter, because this simply isn't true. The right diet will help you regain and protect your health and address your peripheral neuropathy.

The diet we are recommending for those who suffer from peripheral neuropathy ultimately controls inflammation throughout your body. **This type of inflammation affects every organ, tissue, artery, blood vessel, hormone, and cell and, therefore, determines your state of health**.

Studies show that inflammation is the underlying cause of death in America, like heart disease and cancer. It is the root cause of the majority of the degenerative diseases we are facing today.

All grains break down into sugar when digested. Sugar causes an **inflammatory reaction**, particularly in individuals suffering with inflammatory conditions, such as heart disease, arthritis, chronic fatigue, fibromyalgia, neuropathy, and irritable bowel syndrome just to name a few. Removing grains from your diet controls inflammation.

Simply stated, it is impossible to cure many of the diseases that mankind faces without addressing inflammation. There will be no cure for many of the biggest killers unless we make the necessary changes to diet and embark on detoxification. There will, in the end, be no magic pill.

But the fact that there will be no magic pill does not mean that there can't be a sort of magic. By opting for the right approaches to food and treatment, it is possible give your body a break and, in the process, help boost your energy and vitality. It is not magic but science, and the end result is that you'll feel much better.

Our Optimal-Health Eating Plan is a specific diet and a remarkably powerful tool in the fight against peripheral neuropathy. Let's look a bit closer at how this diet works.

THE RIGHT DIET WILL HELP YOU CONTROL INFLAMMATION

The Optimal-Health Eating Plan focuses largely on **removing sugars and everything that turns into sugar**, which would include grains and rice. There are other good reasons to remove rice from your diet as well, such as the fact that most rice is high in arsenic. Next we want to increase the good fats in your diet. What are good fats? Good fats come in the form of olive oil, flaxseed oil, coconut oil, omega-3–rich fish, and fish oils, such as sardines and wild Alaskan salmon.

Following this dietary path allows the diet to do three very important things for you body: remove toxins, regulate hormone function, and decrease inflammation. Ultimately, this new dietary approach will assist your body in the natural healing process. If you give your body the right food and the optimal conditions for healing, some pretty amazing things begin to happen. For example, your body is made up of over seventy trillion cells. When you select the right diet, you power them to work in your benefit. As a result, your body starts to self-regulate its own inflammation.

As you know, every organ, cell, and nerve in your body is affected by inflammation. This also includes your arteries, capillaries, and blood vessels that serve your nerves. When you think about these factors, obviously it only makes sense that inflammation is closely tied to peripheral neuropathy.

Inflammation is the great unsung killer of our time. Most people are unaware of the impact that inflammation plays in their lives and how inflammation contributes to diseases, a range of conditions, slow wound healing, and general pain.

A LOW-INFLAMMATION DIET CONTRIBUTES TO DETOXIFICATION

The second way that a low-inflammation diet helps your body is to contribute to detoxification. Few people realize that detoxification must occur at the cellular level. Nutrients must move in, and toxins must come out in order for cells to be clean and healthy. The cell membrane is the gatekeeper that allows this to occur.

The standard American diet and our toxic environment cause our cell membrane to be inflamed. When the cell membrane becomes inflamed, the above process is hindered. The cells become toxic, and this issue, of course, leads to a wide spectrum of health problems.

Detoxification will help your condition improve and regulate your insulin if you are a diabetic. Insulin is the number-one hormone that needs to be regulated in the systems of those who suffer from diabetic neuropathy.

The four big effects of a low-inflammation diet are:

1. Lowering high triglycerides and cholesterol: if you are a sugar burner and not a fat burner, your body will not store or burn fat normally. As a result, triglyceride levels will become elevated (100 to 135 is normal; >135 is elevated. Optimal total cholesterol levels range from 150 to 200).
2. Lowering high blood pressure: few people realize the key fact that inflammation of the large arteries leads to high blood pressure. Inflammation of the microcirculation leads to peripheral neuropathy and other organ malfunctions. The good news is that a low-inflammation diet works to actually *decrease* inflammation in the body.
3. Lowering high glucose and insulin: once the insulin receptors are burned out, a fasting glucose, insulin test will be elevated. Removing all sugar is the only way to heal the insulin receptors.
4. Weight loss resistance: a low-inflammation diet works for weight-loss resistance because of its effect on hormones and toxins. If you are a person who struggles to lose weight despite what you eat and how much you exercise, a low-inflammation diet, as outlined in this book, is the *only* diet that will work for you.

You want to have triglycerides and cholesterol at optimum level, which means triglycerides at 100 to 135 and optimal cholesterol range should be 150 to 200. Our low-inflammation diet helps to regulate cholesterol and triglycerides and then high blood pressure.

High blood pressure is caused by inflammation of the large arteries. It is very important to note that inflammation in microcirculation is what leads to peripheral neuropathy and other organ malfunctions. In regard to glucose and insulin, once the insulin receptors are burned out, fasting glucose insulin tests will show elevated levels. Removing all sugars is the only way to heal these insulin receptors. As I have stated, a low-inflammation diet is key.

THE FIVE BASICS OF THIS DIET

We must eliminate all sugars and everything that turns to sugar to heal the hormone-insulin-receptor sites and decrease inflammation. You've read a lot about this amazing diet so far in this book. But what exactly does it entail? Let's take a look.

1. NO SUGARS. Yes, no sugars. This includes all sugar forms and artificial sweeteners. Stevia is acceptable.
2. NO GRAINS. And that means even whole, healthy grains are off-limits.
3. NO BAD FATS. Instead of eating bad fats, like those in fried foods, focus on increasing healthy fats, like olive oil and avocado.
4. LIMIT FRUIT. It's important to note that, while fruit should be limited, all berries are fine, such as strawberries, blueberries, blackberries, etc.
5. CHECK YOUR PROTEIN INTAKE. Protein is vital for good health, but so is keeping your protein levels in check.

GETTING THE MOST OUT OF A LOW-INFLAMMATION DIET

Making the decision to transform your diet and embrace different and healthy foods will go a long way toward detoxifying your body, but there are other steps that you also can embrace. At the top of the list are eating foods that are designed to detoxify your body. In the next section, we will explore the foods that you should eat to reduce inflammation, as well as incorporating special foods to detoxify your body.

STEP ONE: ELIMINATE SUGAR

Since grains get turned into sugar, they need to go. As difficult as it may be to give up grains since you have likely eaten them regularly throughout your life, remember that this will make a big difference to your health. You will see positive results on this diet. Remember the issue with sugar is that it not only damages your DNA, but it also triggers inflammation. So, in short, grains and sugar are a double whammy and should be avoided.

The importance of reducing sugar also means keeping an eye on your fruit consumption as well. In general, fruits are loaded with antioxidants, vitamins, and minerals, but they are also high in sugar. Berries—such as blueberries, strawberries, and so forth—are fine, but you will want to limit your consumption of other fruits considerably.

Now, eliminating sugar does *not* mean that you should opt for artificial sweeteners instead. Consuming artificial sweeteners—and they are hiding everywhere—is one of the worst things you can possibly do for your body, period. So don't reach for a diet soda as a way to eat less sugar.

Study after study has shown that artificial sweeteners are extremely bad for your health and will increase your chances of developing a range of diseases. In fact, artificial sweeteners have been linked to everything from a dramatically increased risk of cancer to neurological disorders. Obviously, with this kind of negative track record, the last so-called food you want to consume is anything that contains artificial sweeteners. Just like sugar, artificial sweeteners will also increase inflammation in your body.

STEP TWO: SELECT THE RIGHT KIND OF PROTEIN

Check your protein intake. On average, males should be consuming twenty grams and women fifteen grams of protein in each meal. Just to give you some idea of what this looks like, an egg typically contains seven grams of protein; a piece of meat the size of a deck of cards contains fifteen grams of protein.

Not all protein is created equally. Far too many people are consuming the wrong kinds of protein, and it is killing them. Protein that is loaded down with trans fat (aka bad fats) contributes to inflammation and all the diseases that come with it, such as peripheral neuropathy. Let's look at some of the protein choices that you *should* have in your diet.

HEALTHY PROTEIN CHOICES: NINE KEY FACTS

1. Start reading labels. Choose grass-fed, free-range, cage-free or no-hormone-added protein sources whenever possible.
2. Avoid farm-raised and Atlantic fish. Why? We could dedicate an entire book to the issue of fish and contamination. Farm-raised fish, like salmon, are full of contaminants, such as flame-retardant chemicals, to name just one. Atlantic fish is problematic because it is generally higher in heavy metals, such as mercury and lead, which can damage organs and the brain. Overall, it is best to choose to consume fish in moderation due to mercury levels.
3. Choose cold-water fish, especially, wild Alaskan salmon. The reason that wild Alaskan salmon ranks so high on the list of protein choices is that it is loaded with omega-3 fatty acids. Remember from earlier in the book that omega-3 fatty acids actually fight inflammation exceptionally well. So eating seafood rich in omega-3 fatty acids will work toward making you better.

4. **Sardines are one of nature's more impressive foods.** Since sardines are low on the food chain, they generally have less contamination than other types of fish. Additionally, sardines are very low in calories, high in protein, and also rich in omega-3 fatty acids. If you opt for sardines that are not deboned, you will also get an impressive amount of calcium in every serving.

5. Eggs have received a lot of bad press, but the attitude toward eggs within the medical community is changing. The reason is the simple: **there is a great deal of nutrition in eggs.** By choosing omega-3–enriched eggs, it is possible to boost your omega-3 intake without boosting your calories. This helps to make omega-3–enriched eggs a very savvy choice. Eggs are also an easily digested form of protein.

6. Other animal protein choices—such as chicken, turkey and grass-fed beef—are fine in very small, occasional quantities as so long as they are organic and preferably free-range.

7. **Whey protein has many benefits.** First, it is very low in calories and very high in protein. Studies have also pointed to the fact that whey protein appears to boost the immune system. One exceptional option that is gaining ground is goat-whey protein. The reason that goat dairy products are receiving more attention is due to the fact that growth hormones, excessive antibiotic treatments, and the problems associated with mass dairy farming are generally not present in goat dairy.

8. There are many excellent vegan options when it comes to protein as well. Grounded flaxseeds are extremely high in omega-3 fatty acids, as are walnuts. Nuts are an excellent source of protein, and walnuts rank at the top of the list because they are rich in vitamins, minerals, and omega-3 fatty acids.

9. The time you invest in changing the proteins you eat will make a significant difference in your health and in addressing your peripheral neuropathy. Unhealthy protein choices, such as fried foods and those heavy in trans fats, cause inflammation. Whereas the protein choices we have outlined above will actually help your body fight

inflammation, and that means your body's natural healing mechanism will begin to help you.

ADDITIONAL PROTEIN OPTIONS

— raw cheeses
— cottage cheese
— ricotta cheese
— game birds, such as duck, goose, grouse and pheasant
— venison
— small servings of wild cold-water fish, such as mahimahi and mackerel

STEP THREE: SELECT THE RIGHT KINDS OF HEALTHY FAT

Just as selecting the right proteins can transform your health, the same also holds true for selecting the right fats. Contrary to common perception, fats don't make you fat. The idea that all fat is bad and will harm you has, in fact, done a tremendous amount of serious damage to society's collective health and well-being. Fat is not like smoking. There is no good smoking versus bad smoking, but there are good fats.

The bottom line is that your body absolutely needs fat to stay healthy, but it needs the right kind of fats. Right now, far too many people are consuming the wrong kinds of fats, thanks to the fast-food and processed-food industries. As we can see from the obesity epidemic, the wrong kinds of fat do contribute to making people very unhealthy.

Your cell membrane needs healthy fats, so choose healthy fats, like raw nuts and seeds, walnuts, almonds, and cashews. These types of choices are great and very healthy for you. Olive oil, avocados, coconut milk, and fish oils, such as cod-liver oil, are the kinds of healthy fats that you need.

Eggs are also good, and even a very small amount of organic butter is fine in moderation.

TEN BEST SOURCES OF FAT

1. Nuts, such as walnuts, have high omega-3 fatty-acid levels.
2. Seeds, such as sunflower or sesame seeds, are a great source of healthy natural fat.
3. Wild Alaskan salmon is a healthy-fat superstar.
4. Sardines are low in calories and abundant in omega-3 fatty acids.
5. Omega-3–enriched eggs.
6. Studies have shown that olive oil works to fight inflammation throughout the body.
7. Avocados are one of nature's most impressive foods. This member of the fruit family has an abundance of healthy fat and will improve your health.
8. Fish oils are a fantastic source of omega-3 fatty acids. Cod-liver oil is a great fish oil pick, but it is important to opt for a higher grade option. The reason that you should only consume higher-grade fish oils (ones that have been purified) is due to heavy metals, such as mercury, that can become concentrated in fish. Any cod-liver oil you take should be purified.
9. There are other alternatives to cod-liver oil, such as fish oils made from sardines and anchovies. Sardines and anchovies are small fish, so they are lower on the food chain than most other fish. As a result, they make excellent fish oil, as they are naturally low in heavy metals and other contaminants. Despite that, however, it is still vital that you only take fish-oil supplements that have been purified.
10. There is one fish-oil supplement that is the exception to the purification rule, and that is krill oil. Krill rank very low on the food chain, and this means they, of course, have very low levels of contamination.

Krill oil is also harvested from the waters off of Antarctica, which also contributes to low contamination levels. Increasingly, krill oil is seen as an excellent way to fight inflammation.

ADDITIONAL EXCELLENT SOURCES OF GOOD FAT

— Raw nuts, such as almonds, cashews, pecans, and macadamia nuts
— Raw seeds, such as sesame and sunflower seeds
— Nut butters
— Coconut milk, oil, flakes, or spread
— Grape-seed oil
— Hemp powder
— Hemp oil (three to one ratio)
— Full fat, plain yogurt
— Probiotic rich kefir, which is low in calories and high in protein and calcium

You may have noticed that there is some overlap between the healthy protein and healthy fat choices; this is due to the omega-3 fatty-acid factor. Since omega-3 fatty acids fight inflammation, the foods that are both excellent sources of protein and high in omega-3 are easy choices for both lists. The fact that some foods are on both lists is also a strong clue that these are key foods you should consider building part of your diet around.

THE FATS YOU SHOULD BE *AVOIDING*

Be sure to always avoid hydrogenated and partially hydrogenated oils—such as cottonseed oil, soybean oil, and vegetable oils—and trans fats, such as margarine and synthetic butters. Rancid vegetable oils, such as corn oil, canola oil, or those labeled simply vegetable oil are unfortunately located in practically every bread, cracker, cookie, and boxed food.

STEP FOUR: ORGANIC VEGETABLES

Is organic food worth the investment? The short answer is yes. Organic vegetables have fewer toxins in them and better vitamin content.

Nonorganic fruits and vegetables can receive a lot of pesticide exposure. What further complicates this issue is the fact that pesticide levels and the number of different types of pesticides used on nonorganic fruits and vegetables vary wildly depending upon the fruit or vegetable in question. Soft fruits, such as strawberries and peaches, for example, receive much more pesticide exposure than an avocado. Opting for organic produce is a must, as it will help detoxify your body.

HIGH-FIBER CARBOHYDRATE (VEGETABLES) CHOICES

Choose organic when possible. Remember the best carbohydrate choices are these vegetables, due to high fiber content and low glycemic action.

Eat as much of the following foods as you desire:

arugula	asparagus
bamboo shoots	bean sprouts
beet greens	bell peppers (red, yellow, and green)
broad beans	broccoli
brussels sprouts	cabbage
cassava	cauliflower
celery	chayote fruit

chicory

chives

collard greens

coriander

cucumber

dandelion greens

eggplant

endive

fennel

garlic

ginger root

green beans

hearts of palm

jicama (raw)

jalapeño peppers

kale

kohlrabi

lettuce

mushrooms

mustard greens

onions

parsley

radishes

radicchio

snap beans

snow peas

shallots

spinach

spaghetti squash

summer squash

Swiss chard

turnip greens

watercress

CARBOHYDRATE CHOICES IN MODERATION

The following choices are also fine unless you are weight-loss resistant or trying to lose weight. Otherwise, consume as much of these as you wish:

artichokes

yellow beans

tomatoes

leeks

okra

pumpkin

legumes

turnip

adzuki beans

black beans

chickpeas

lima beans

great northern beans

French beans

kidney beans

navy beans

mung beans	lentils
pinto beans	split peas
white beans	squash (acorn, butternut, and winter)
quinoa and buckwheat (in extreme moderation)	

LOW-GI (GLYCEMIC INDEX) FRUIT CHOICES IN MODERATION ONLY!

Once again, when you are selecting fruit, choose organic when possible. If weight loss is a concern, eat fruit in extreme moderation.

Low-GI fruit choices include berries (blackberries, blueberries, boysen-berries, elderberries, gooseberries, loganberries, raspberries, strawberries), avocados, lemons, limes, kiwi, and Granny Smith apples. Fruits are best con-sumed within one hour of exercise and with proteins, such as grass-fed whey protein.

LOW-FIBER CARBOHYDRATES TO ELIMINATE

The following list of carbohydrates offers high and moderate glycemic action with little fiber to regulate. As a result, they will turn to sugar in your body very quickly.

barley	brown rice
millet	rye
semolina	steel-cut oats
tapioca	whole-grain breads
cooked cereals	bulgur
spelt	ak-mak crackers

whole grains
Ezekiel bread
whole-grain tortillas
sprouted grains

Wasa crackers
amaranth
wild rice

KEY SUGAR FACTS

— Refined sugar weakens the immune system.
— Refined sugar *damages DNA!*
— Sugar promotes yeast growth in the body.
— One can of soda has between nine and eleven teaspoons of sugar.
— Sugar is hiding in places where you would never expect to find it, such as bread.
— Processed foods and fast foods are usually loaded with sugar.
— So-called sports drinks and energy drinks are often loaded not just with sugar but also with artificial sweeteners and a range of harmful additives, such as dyes and colorings. In short, you should avoid these drinks.
— Diet soda may not have sugar, but what it does have in the form of chemicals and artificial sweeteners is just as bad if not worse for your health.
— Today Americans consume an average of 120 pounds of sugar per year, per person, compared to five pounds per year per family in the early 1900s.
— Look at the sugar content on labels. Anything with "ose" at the end is sugar, and that means avoid it.

The sugar found in dates, fresh or canned corn, beets, and lactose (lactose is a sugar found in milk, so avoid milk) raw whole milk, rice, and almond milk are fine in moderation.

SUGAR RULES TO LIVE (BETTER) BY: TEN FORMS OF SUGAR TO AVOID

— corn syrup
— fructose
— honey
— sucrose
— maltodextrin
— dextrose
— molasses
— fruit juice
— sweetened brown-rice syrup
— maple syrup (Grade B is fine, but in extreme moderation only)

One more thought on sugar. Sugar can be found in a lot of foods and condiments, and I understand it will be impossible to avoid this all together. Understand that your sugar content must be limited to the least amount possible to achieve the best results. Ultimately, the less sugar you eat the better.

If you are feeling weak or fatigued on this diet, you need to eat more frequently. Don't turn to sugar, as the energy boost sugar will give you is very short-lived. Snack on nuts, seeds, berries, and some high-quality protein between meals to avoid drops in your energy levels.

Stop eating grains until normal glucose and weight are reached, as prescribed in this diet. It will take several days to lower your insulin levels. In the meantime, high insulin levels will cause symptoms, such as dizziness, confusion, headaches, and a general ill feeling.

If you are continuing to feel light-headed and dizzy on this diet, this could also be a sign of your blood pressure improving. As a result, a decrease in your blood pressure medication may be in order. Talk to your primary-care physician about lowering your dose if not eliminating it from your routine.

I explain to my patients that it is not my position to take them off of their medication. That means that whatever doctor put you on a medication is whom you should speak to about adjusting your dose and eliminating it from your regimen.

ADDITIONAL TIPS FOR ADDRESSING LIGHT-HEADEDNESS AND DIZZINESS

— Eating every two hours can help minimize unpleasant symptoms during this transition.

— Eating four to six meals a day is better for weight loss, even after your system adjusts.

— Eating more frequently has shown to normalize blood sugars and sustain energy.

CHAPTER ELEVEN

LIVING WITH OPTIMAL HEALTH

In order to stay well and maintain your new healthy weight and lifestyle, you may have to make some major life changes. Switching over one's diet can be difficult, but what I hear every day from patients is that feeling better, having more energy, sleeping better, and having less pain and numbness makes it worthwhile. More than likely, you will see a major improvement in your peripheral-neuropathy symptoms as a result of the guidelines I've described in this book.

Yet, even with all of these positives, I realize that it can be tough to give up the foods that you love and crave. Let's take a look at a couple of ways that you can keep your sanity while switching over to a new and better diet.

TIP ONE: NEW RECIPES

New recipes that incorporate many of the healthy ingredients you should be eating will help you keep your sanity. If you are like most people, new flavors can go a very long way toward brightening your day. Experiment with spices and fresh herbs to keep your meals interesting.

TIP TWO: KEEP A JOURNAL NOTING HOW MUCH BETTER YOU FEEL

The low-inflammation diet featured in this book can and will help you feel better. One way of keeping your motivation levels up when switching over from your current diet to a low-inflammation one is to literally make notes on how your energy levels are increasing and your pain levels are decreasing. When your willpower starts to weaken, take a look at your journal, and remember that you've dramatically improved how you feel.

TIP THREE: VACATION MEALS

Why not give yourself something to look forward to during the week? There is nothing wrong with a "vacation meal" every now and again. After all, you need to have something to look forward to in the weeks ahead. Vacation meals are allowed after your first ten weeks of care here in the office.

A vacation meal consists of eating anything your heart desires for one meal (breakfast, lunch, or dinner) once a week. For example, in any given week, you can have pancakes for breakfast one day, cheeseburgers for lunch one day, and pizza for dinner one night. The key to all of this is to be eating according to the low-inflammation diet for the rest of your meals and snacks. But it's OK to take a break every now and then.

YOU CAN CONQUER PERIPHERAL NEUROPATHY

Building a new diet can help you build a new life. That might sound a little too easy to be true, but the facts are that a new approach to food and how you eat will transform your health and, in the process, address your peripheral neuropathy. The fact of the matter is that peripheral neuropathy could have more serious consequences, and that means you need to take action.

Traditional approaches to peripheral neuropathy don't work to fix the problem but instead simply place a bandage on the disease. Unfortunately, that bandage comes in the form of pharmaceutical pain-relief drug options that can have profoundly negative impacts on one's life. This is why it is so important to find an approach, like the one outlined in this book, that works to address peripheral neuropathy.

Millions of people suffer from peripheral neuropathy. This ailment negatively impacts quality of life for countless individuals. In short, the current mainstream approach toward *treating* peripheral neuropathy is nothing short of madness.

If you want a healthier life, one where you continue to enjoy everyday living and your mobility, you will want to find an approach to treating your peripheral neuropathy that really works. By opting for the right alternative treatments and selecting a new approach to your diet, you will see dramatic improvements.

There are approaches that really do work. I have highlighted many of them in this book. Ultimately, there is no reason whatsoever that you should become a statistic; you just need to take action.

SUCCESS STORIES

Before coming to Dr. Straw's office, I was experiencing tingling, numbness, and burning pain in my hands and feet, and pain medication only minimized and masked the pain.

Since starting care, I have noticed a tremendous improvement so that I no longer have burning pain, and I DO NOT REQUIRE any of my pain medication! My quality of life is so much BETTER! I am pain-free and sleeping through the night. I am very grateful to all the doctors and staff for their support.

Barbara Beckman, RN, Fullerton, California

Over five years, I've had two back surgeries and physical therapy. I've also seen a neurologist, but he couldn't help me. It got to a point where I had to leave my medical practice as an anesthesiologist because I couldn't mobilize myself in the operating room due to problems with the sense of touch in my feet. I couldn't see myself going through life wondering how much this could progress and whether anything could stop it.

Since I started the Straw Protocol, I have regained my balance, which is very important to me. This treatment is the only thing I have read about that I find credible. I am so happy I did this!

Joseph Warpinski, MD, Mission Viejo, California

Before I came to Dr. Straw's office, I was experiencing numbness in my feet, loss of balance, and difficulty walking. Now after treatment, I have much more feeling back in my feet, so driving is no longer a concern, and my balance has improved. I'm also able to go to the gym now and exercise more.

Bill Covey, retired president, Huntington Memorial Hospital

Since starting the Straw Protocol, I've noticed great improvement all around: less numbness and sensitivity in my feet. It feels like both hands and feet are waking up in a lot less pain! Before starting treatment, my balance was terrible; I could not walk with one foot in front of the other. Now I can walk heel to toe without any assistance. I am now more mobile and feel a lot safer walking (I balance better). I have more energy because of the eating plan. It has helped me be more active, along with the help of the treatment.

Rex D., Corona, California

I am able to walk without having to rely on my cane, which is an amazing feeling. My balance is so much better; I am no longer worried that I may fall. I am also dancing again, and I never thought I would be able to do that again!

Jackie B., Redlands, California

I have more energy. I am able to do my gardening for a long period of time. I am enjoying walking with my daughter, and I can keep up with her. I am now planning a vacation! I am not afraid of the walking; I anticipate the challenge!

Marjorie S., Riverside, California

Before coming to Dr. Straw's office, I was experiencing numbness in both my feet, and they were so icy cold that they burned all the time. My balance was also very poor. I was unable to rise from a sitting position without assistance, and it would take a minute before I regained feeling in my feet. Since starting care, I have noticed my numbness is almost completely gone. I now have feeling in my feet that I have not felt in over twenty years. I can now tell the difference between hot and cold sensations. I am able to rise from sitting without assistance now, and I am no longer using my cane.

Marci D., Rancho Cucamonga, California

Five weeks ago, I couldn't walk one block without severe pain. I've lost thirty-two pounds in thirty-five days. I now walk one and a half miles and bike seven miles a day.

Jeffery T., Fullerton, California

Before coming to Dr. Straw's office, I was starting to lose all hope. I was experiencing extreme pain in my right leg. I was unable to even touch my lower right leg or exercise. Since starting care, my ankle is nowhere near as cold, and the pain is much better. I'm able enjoy life again. Thank You!

Alexis B, Anaheim, California

I knew after the second treatment that God had sent me to the right place. Treatment has strengthened my hands and feet. I can now use my hands to put on my jewelry, pick up small items, and hold things without the fear of dropping them. I have also improved my typing ability. I can now stand because of the use of my toes to anchor my body. I no longer have to hold onto walls or look for a shopping cart to lean on to help me walk. I noticed I am now parking farther away from the store because I can walk without the fear of falling. My balance has greatly improved. My greatest test was when I went to Las Vegas for a meeting. I was able to walk the length of the MGM Hotel without stopping, keeping up with the crowd. If I had not received treatments before I left, I would probably have had to stay in my hotel room. My body is so relaxed now, every night I sleep very well.

Arlene D., Costa Mesa, California

PART TWO

OPTIMAL-
HEALTH
EATING PLAN

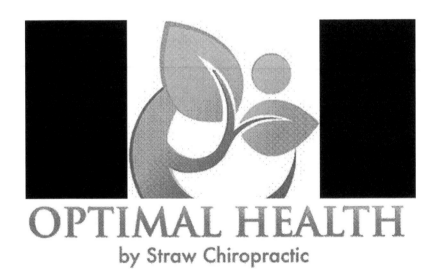

IMPORTANT NOTICE

The Optimal-Health Eating Plan is intended for patients without dietary restrictions or under any other eating plans prescribed by your doctor. If you have been advised on your diet or are currently on an eating plan prescribed by your doctor, do not alter that existing eating plan until consulting with him/her or one of our physicians.

NOTICE TO PATIENTS: If you have any dietary restrictions, medical conditions, or are on medications for which your doctor has prescribed a dietary plan, do not begin this eating plan until consulting with a physician.

Ingredients
A grocery list is provided for each weekly menu. Use the corresponding grocery list as a checklist. Most ingredients will repeat from one week to another. You will most likely have leftover ingredients from your previous purchase and will not have to buy more.

Most ingredients can be found at your local supermarket. For ingredients that are hard to find, suggestions are listed below on the grocery list.

Vegetarians
Vegetarian recipes are marked with a green leaf next to the recipe's name.

Snacks
Snacks are not provided on the weekly menu. Snacks are optional. You can make your own snacks with the recipes provided under the snack tab, or you

can purchase them in stores. A list of snacks you can purchase in stores if you do not wish not to make your own is provided under the snack tab.

ATTENTION: PATIENTS ON WARFARIN (COUMADIN)

Vitamin K can lessen the effectiveness of warfarin (Coumadin). It's important to pay attention to what you eat while on warfarin. It's also important to be consistent in how much vitamin K you get daily. Eating small amounts of foods that are rich in vitamin K shouldn't cause a problem. Avoid large amounts of kale, spinach, Brussels sprouts, parsley, collard greens, mustard greens, chard, and green tea.

Also avoid or drink only small amounts of cranberry juice and alcohol when taking warfarin.

Recipes that contain the listed ingredients above are marked with a red heart next to the recipe's name. Please replace these with an alternative recipe of your choice. If you wish to use these recipes, you may replace the listed ingredients with other vegetables of choice or reduce the amount.

WEEKLY MENU OPTIONS
AND
GROCERY LISTS

WEEK ONE

	Breakfast	Lunch	Dinner
Monday	Baked Eggs in Prosciutto-Filled Portobello Mushroom Caps	Beef and Butternut Squash Stew with Rosemary and Balsamic Vinegar	Chicken Broccoli Alfredo
Tuesday	🌿 Scrambled Eggs with Basil and Walnuts	Fish Tacos	Lemon, Garlic, and Herb Pork Chops
Wednesday	🌿 No-Oat Oatmeal	Pork-Fried Cauliflower Rice	Zucchini and Ground Beef
Thursday	Kitchen Hash	Tuna-Salad Celery Boats with Avocado and Dill	Hatch Chile Meatballs
Friday	🖤 Grilled Garlic Mushrooms with Bacon	🌿 Turkey Lettuce-Wrap Tacos with Chilies, Cumin, Cilantro, Lime, and Tomato-Avocado Salsa	Herb-Spinach Chicken Burgers
Saturday	🖤 Zucchini Pancake Breakfast Tower	🖤 Vegetable Cauliflower Rice	🖤 Simple Bacon and Spinach–Stuffed Chicken
Sunday	🌿 Pumpkin Porridge	🖤 Ground-Beef Skillet	Easy Chicken Dinner in 1...2...3

89

WEEK ONE GROCERY LIST

SEASONINGS	OTHERS	PRODUCE
		__ Medium to Large Portobello Mushroom
__ Black Pepper	__ Almond Milk (Unsweetened)	__ Parsley
__ Salt	__ Coconut Milk	__ Thyme
__ Ground Cinnamon	__ Pumpkin Puree	__ Fresh Basil
__ Ground Nutmeg	__ Diced, Jarred Roasted Red Pepper	__ Banana
__ Ground Ginger	__ Low-Sodium Beef Broth or Beef Stock	__ Fresh Berries
__ Garlic Powder	__ Coconut Amino	__ Yellow and Red Bell Peppers
__ Onion Powder	__ Canned Tuna	__ Yellow and Red Onion
__ Vanilla Extract	__ Mayonnaise	__ Spinach
__ Allspice	__ Olive Oil	__ Butternut Squash
__ Sea Salt	__ Coconut Oil	__ Rosemary
__ NuNatural Stevia	__ Dijon Mustard	__ Avocado
__ Balsamic Vinegar	__ Clarified Butter	__ Lime and Lemon
__ Dried Oregano	__ Almond Flour (Whole Foods, Mothers Market, Sprouts)	__ Fresh Cilantro
__ Dill	__ Coconut Flour (Whole Foods, Mothers Market, Sprouts)	__ Tomatoes
__ Ground Cumin	__ Almond Butter	__ Cauliflower
__ Ground Cayenne Pepper		__ Carrots

__ Dried Thyme

__ Dried Basil

__ Paprika

DRIED INGREDIENTS

__ Walnuts

__ Pecans

__ Ground Flaxseed

__ Pumpkin Seeds

MEATS

__ Farm-Fresh Eggs

__ Prosciutto

__ Chorizo

__ Chicken Breast

__ Bacon (Turkey)

__ Beef Tri-Tip

__ Mahimahi (or Salmon)

__ Pork

__ Ground Turkey

__ Lean Ground Beef

__ Pork Chops

__ Ground Chicken

__ Garlic Cloves

__ Celery Sticks

__ Green Chilies

__ Green Onions

__ Jalapeno

__ Romaine

__ Asparagus

__ Radish

__ Spaghetti Squash

__ Broccoli

__ Zucchini

WEEK TWO

	Breakfast	Lunch	Dinner
Monday	Chicken Chorizo "No-Potato" Hash	Beef Stew	Grilled Salmon with Avocado Salsa
Tuesday	Tuna and Egg Sandwich	Cauliflower Tabbouleh	Grilled Chicken with Greek Sweet Potatoes
Wednesday	Dijon Egg and Veggie Scramble	Herb Turkey Burgers with Zucchini Buns	Simple Herb-Crusted Salmon
Thursday	Kitchen Hash	Tuna-Salad Celery Boats with Avocado and Dill	Hatch Chile Meatballs
Friday	Breakfast Zucchini Pancakes	Pork-Fried Cauliflower Rice	Roasted Garlic, Spinach, and Mushroom–Stuffed Pork Chops
Saturday	Breakfast Burrito	Zucchini Pesto Roll-Ups	Pork Burgers
Sunday	Granola Cereal	Pepper Poppers	Simple Bacon and Spinach–Stuffed Chicken

WEEK TWO GROCERY LIST

SEASONINGS	OTHERS	PRODUCE
__ Salt	__ Olive Oil	__ Red and Yellow Onion
__ Pepper	__ Canned Tuna	__ Cilantro
__ Vanilla	__ Almond Flour (Whole Foods, Mothers Market, Sprouts)	__ Zucchini
__ Sage	__ Dijon Mustard	__ Red Chili Peppers
__ Ground Fennel	__ Honey	__ Bell Peppers (Red, Yellow, and Green)
__ Garlic Powder	__ Almond Butter	__ Sweet Potatoes
__ Dried Oregano	__ Coconut Oil	__ Carrots
__ Red-Pepper Flakes	__ Beef Stock or Beef Broth	__ Green Peas
__ Ground Coriander	__ White-Wine Vinegar	__ Green Onion
__ Cumin	__ Coconut Flour (Whole Foods, Mothers Market, Sprouts)	__ Spinach
__ Paprika Powder		__ Tomatoes and Cherry Tomatoes
__ Onion Powder		__ Avocado
__ Dried Thyme		__ Celery
		__ Rosemary
		__ Thyme
		__ Cauliflower

DRIED INGREDIENTS

__ Pecans

__ Almonds

__ Dried Cranberries

__ Shredded Coconut

__ Walnuts

MEATS

__ Chorizo

__ Chicken breast

__ Egg

__ Ham

__ Beef Tri-Tip

__ Ground Pork

__ Ground Turkey

__ Italian Sausage

__ Salmon

__ Pork Chops

__ Ground Chicken

__ Bacon (Turkey)

__ Parsley

__ Mint

__ Lemon and Lime

__ Garlic

__ Oregano

__ Basil

__ Baby Sweet Peppers

__ Kale

__ Arugula

__ Portobello Button Mushrooms

WEEK THREE

	Breakfast	Lunch	Dinner
Monday	Brussels Sprout and Spinach Truffle Frittata	Spicy Redfish Stew	Zucchini and Ground Beef
Tuesday	Easy Breakfast Scramble	Lemon and Almond Cauliflower Rice	Chicken Piccata
Wednesday	Roasted Eggplant Stacks	Chicken Fajita Salad	Grilled Salmon with Avocado Salsa
Thursday	Porridge with Berries	Creamy Zucchini Pasta with Shrimp	Zucchini Fettuccine Alfredo
Friday	Salmon and Zucchini Fritters	Vegetable Cauliflower Rice	Simple Herb-Crusted Salmon
Saturday	Scrambled Eggs with Mushrooms and Pine Nuts	Grain-Free Salmon Rolls	Pork Burgers
Sunday	Asparagus and Basil Omelets	Fajitas	Crispy-Skin Salmon

WEEK THREE GROCERY LIST

SEASONINGS	OTHERS	PRODUCE
__ Garlic Powder	__ Truffle Oil	__ Brussels Sprouts
__ Paprika	__ Clarified Butter	__ Fresh Spinach
__ Salt	__ Jarred Sundried Tomatoes	__ Garlic Cloves
__ Pepper	__ Olive Oil	__ Avocado
__ Herbes de Provence	__ Balsamic Vinegar	__ Parsley
__ Sea Salt	__ Coconut Oil	__ Sweet Potatoes
__ Red-Pepper Flakes	__ Almond Flour (Whole Foods, Mothers Market, Sprouts)	__ Yellow and Red Onions
__ Cumin	__ Capers	__ Bell Peppers
__ Oregano	__ Chicken Stock (Broth)	__ Mushrooms
	__ Coconut Cream	__ Eggplant
	__ Coconut Water	__ Tomatoes
		__ Berries
		__ Zucchini
		__ Dill
DRIED INGREDIENTS	MEATS	__ Asparagus
		__ Basil
__ Shredded, Unsweetened Coconut	__ Ground Beef	__ Sage
__ Raw Walnuts	__ Eggs	__ Chives
__ Sliced Almonds	__ Smoked Salmon	__ Cilantro
__ Raw Pepitas (Shelled Pumpkin Seeds)	__ Sausage	__ Lemon and Lime

WEEKLY MENU OPTIONS AND GROCERY LISTS

__ Ground Flaxseed

__ Almonds

__ Choice of Fish

__ Chicken Breast

__ Shrimp

__ Salmon Fillet (Skin on)

__ Cauliflower

__ Red-Leaf or Romaine Lettuce

__ Tomatoes

__ Avocado

__ Large Cucumber

__ One Peach

__ One Small Mango

__ Jalapeno

__ Celery

WEEK FOUR

	Breakfast	Lunch	Dinner
Monday	Baked Eggs in Prosciutto-Filled Portobello Mushroom Caps	Beef and Butternut Squash Stew with Rosemary and Balsamic Vinegar	Chicken Broccoli Alfredo
Tuesday	🌿 Scrambled Eggs with Basil and Walnuts	Fish Tacos	Lemon, Garlic, and Herb Pork Chops
Wednesday	🌿 No-Oat Oatmeal	Pork-Fried Cauliflower Rice	Zucchini and Ground Beef
Thursday	Kitchen Hash	Tuna-Salad Celery Boats with Avocado and Dill	Hatch Chile Meatballs
Friday	💜 Grilled Garlic Mushrooms with Bacon	🌿 Turkey Lettuce-Wrap Tacos with Chilies, Cumin, Cilantro, Lime and Tomato-Avocado Salsa	Herb Spinach Chicken Burgers
Saturday	💜 Zucchini Pancake Breakfast Tower	💜 Vegetable Cauliflower Rice	💜 Simple Bacon and Spinach–Stuffed Chicken
Sunday	🌿 Pumpkin Porridge	💜 Ground-Beef Skillet	Easy Chicken Dinner in 1...2...3

WEEK FOUR GROCERY LIST

SEASONINGS	OTHERS	PRODUCE
		__ Medium to Large Portobello Mushroom
__ Black Pepper	__ Almond Milk (unsweetened)	__ Parsley
__ Salt	__ Coconut Milk	__ Thyme
__ Ground Cinnamon	__ Pumpkin Puree	__ Fresh Basil
__ Ground Nutmeg	__ Diced, Jarred Roasted Red Pepper	__ Banana
__ Ground Ginger	__ Low-Sodium Beef Broth or Beef Stock	__ Fresh berries
__ Garlic Powder	__ Coconut Amino	__ Yellow and Red Bell Peppers
__ Onion Powder	__ Canned Tuna	__ Yellow and Red Onion
__ Vanilla Extract	__ Mayonnaise	__ Spinach
__ Allspice	__ Olive Oil	__ Butternut Squash
__ Sea Salt	__ Coconut Oil	__ Rosemary
__ NuNatural Stevia	__ Dijon Mustard	__ Avocado
__ Balsamic Vinegar	__ Clarified Butter	__ Lime and Lemon
__ Dried Oregano	__ Almond Flour (Whole Foods, Mothers Market, Sprouts)	__ Fresh Cilantro
__ Dill	__ Coconut Flour (Whole Foods, Mothers Market, Sprouts)	__ Tomatoes
__ Ground Cumin	__ Almond Butter	__ Cauliflower
__ Ground Cayenne Pepper		__ Carrots

__ Dried Thyme

__ Dried Basil

__ Paprika

DRIED INGREDIENTS

__ Walnuts

__ Pecans

__ Ground Flaxseed

__ Pumpkin Seeds

MEATS

__ Farm-Fresh Eggs

__ Prosciutto

__ Chorizo

__ Chicken Breast

__ Bacon (Turkey)

__ Beef Tri-Tip

__ Mahimahi (or Salmon)

__ Pork

__ Ground Turkey

__ Lean Ground Beef

__ Pork Chops

__ Ground Chicken

__ Garlic Cloves

__ Celery Sticks

__ Green Chilies

__ Green Onions

__ Jalapeno

__ Romaine

__ Asparagus

__ Radish

__ Spaghetti Squash

__ Broccoli

__ Zucchini

WEEK FIVE

	Breakfast	Lunch	Dinner
Monday	Chicken Chorizo "No-Potato" Hash	Beef Stew	Grilled Salmon with Avocado Salsa
Tuesday	Tuna and Egg Sandwich	Cauliflower Tabbouleh	Grilled Chicken with Greek Sweet Potatoes
Wednesday	Dijon Egg and Veggie Scramble	Herb Turkey Burgers with Zucchini Buns	Simple Herb-Crusted Salmon
Thursday	Kitchen Hash	Tuna-Salad Celery Boats with Avocado and Dill	Hatch Chile Meatballs
Friday	Breakfast Zucchini Pancakes	Pork-Fried Cauliflower Rice	Roasted Garlic, Spinach, and Mushroom–Stuffed Pork Chops
Saturday	Breakfast Burrito	Zucchini Pesto Roll-Ups	Pork Burgers
Sunday	Granola Cereal	Pepper Poppers	Simple Bacon and Spinach-Stuffed Chicken

WEEK FIVE GROCERY LIST

SEASONINGS	OTHERS	PRODUCE
__ Salt	__ Olive Oil	__ Red and Yellow Onion
__ Pepper	__ Canned Tuna	__ Cilantro
__ Vanilla	__ Almond Flour (Whole Foods, Mothers Market, Sprouts)	__ Zucchini
__ Sage	__ White-Wine Vinegar	__ Red Chili Pepper
__ Ground Fennel	__ Honey	__ Bell Peppers (Red, Yellow, and Green)
__ Garlic Powder	__ Almond Butter	__ Sweet Potatoes
__ Dried Oregano	__ Coconut Oil	__ Carrots
__ Red-Pepper Flakes	__ Beef Stock or Beef Broth	__ Green Peas
__ Ground Coriander	__ Dijon Mustard	__ Green Onion
__ Cumin	__ Coconut Flour (Whole Foods, Mothers Market, Sprouts)	__ Spinach
__ Paprika Powder		__ Tomatoes and Cherry Tomatoes
__ Onion Powder		__ Avocado
__ Dried Thyme		__ Celery
		__ Rosemary
		__ Thyme
		__ Cauliflower

DRIED INGREDIENTS	MEATS	
		__ Parsley
		__ Mint
__ Pecans	__ Chorizo	__ Lemon and Lime
__ Almonds	__ Chicken Breast	__ Garlic
__ Dried Cranberries	__ Eggs	__ Oregano
__ Shredded Coconut	__ Ham	__ Basil
__ Walnut	__ Beef Tri-Tip	__ Baby Sweet Peppers
	__ Ground Pork	__ Kale
	__ Ground Turkey	__ Arugula
	__ Italian Sausage	__ Portobello Button Mushrooms
	__ Salmon	
	__ Pork Chops	
	__ Ground Chicken	
	__ Bacon (Turkey)	

WEEK SIX

	Breakfast	Lunch	Dinner
Monday	BrusselsSprout and Spinach Truffle Frittata	Spicy Redfish Stew	Zucchini and Ground Beef
Tuesday	Easy Breakfast Scramble	Lemon and Almond Cauliflower Rice	Chicken Piccata
Wednesday	Roasted Eggplant Stacks	Chicken Fajita Salad	Grilled Salmon with Avocado Salsa
Thursday	Porridge with Berries	Creamy Zucchini Pasta with Shrimp	Zucchini Fettuccine Alfredo
Friday	Salmon and Zucchini Fritters	Vegetable Cauliflower Rice	Simple Herb-Crusted Salmon
Saturday	Scrambled Eggs with Mushrooms and Pine Nuts	Grain-Free Salmon Rolls	Pork Burgers
Sunday	Asparagus and Basil Omelets	Fajitas	Crispy-Skin Salmon

WEEK SIX GROCERY LIST

SEASONINGS	OTHERS	PRODUCE
__ Garlic Powder	__ Truffle Oil	__ Brussels Sprouts
__ Paprika	__ Clarified Butter	__ Fresh Spinach
__ Salt	__ Jarred Sundried Tomatoes	__ Garlic Cloves
__ Pepper	__ Olive Oil	__ Avocado
__ Herbes de Provence	__ Balsamic Vinegar	__ Parsley
__ Sea Salt	__ Coconut Oil	__ Sweet Potatoes
__ Red-Pepper Flakes	__ Almond Flour (Whole Foods, Mothers Market, Sprouts)	__ Yellow and Red Onions
__ Cumin	__ Capers	__ Bell Pepper
__ Oregano	__ Chicken Stock (Broth)	__ Mushrooms
	__ Coconut Cream	__ Eggplant
	__ Coconut Water	__ Tomatoes
		__ Berries
		__ Zucchini
		__ Dill

DRIED INGREDIENTS	MEATS	__ Asparagus
		__ Basil
__ Shredded, Unsweetened Coconut	__ Ground Beef	__ Sage
__ Raw Walnuts	__ Eggs	__ Chives
__ Sliced Almonds	__ Smoked Salmon	__ Cilantro

NEUROPATHY

__ Raw Pepitas (Shelled Pumpkin Seeds)

__ Ground Flaxseed

__ Almonds

__ Sausage

__ Choice of Fish

__ Chicken Breast

__ Shrimp

__ Salmon Fillet (Skin On)

__ Lemon and Lime

__ Cauliflower

__ Red-Leaf or Romaine Lettuce

__ Tomatoes

__ Avocado

__ Large Cucumber

__ One Peach

__ One Small Mango

__ Jalapeno

__ Celery

WEEK SEVEN

	Breakfast	Lunch	Dinner
Monday	Baked Eggs in Prosciutto-Filled Portobello Mushroom Caps	Beef and Butternut Squash Stew with Rosemary and Balsamic Vinegar	Chicken Broccoli Alfredo
Tuesday	Scrambled Eggs with Basil and Walnuts	Fish Tacos	Lemon, Garlic, and Herb Pork Chops
Wednesday	No-Oat Oatmeal	Pork-Fried Cauliflower Rice	Zucchini and Ground Beef
Thursday	Kitchen Hash	Tuna-Salad Celery Boats with Avocado and Dill	Hatch Chile Meatballs
Friday	Grilled Garlic Mushrooms with Bacon	Turkey Lettuce-Wrap Tacos with Chilies, Cumin, Cilantro, Lime, and Tomato-Avocado Salsa	Herb Spinach Chicken Burgers
Saturday	Zucchini Pancake Breakfast Tower	Vegetable Cauliflower Rice	Simple Bacon and Spinach–Stuffed Chicken
Sunday	Pumpkin Porridge	Ground-Beef Skillet	Easy Chicken Dinner in 1...2...3

WEEK SEVEN GROCERY LIST

SEASONINGS	OTHERS	PRODUCE
		__ Medium to Large Portobello Mushroom
__ Black Pepper	__ Almond Milk (Unsweetened)	__ Parsley
__ Salt	__ Coconut Milk	__ Thyme
__ Ground Cinnamon	__ Pumpkin Puree	__ Fresh Basil
__ Ground Nutmeg	__ Diced, Jarred Roasted Red Pepper	__ Banana
__ Ground Ginger	__ Low-Sodium Beef Broth or Beef Stock	__ Fresh Berries
__ Garlic Powder	__ Coconut Amino	__ Yellow and Red Bell Peppers
__ Onion Powder	__ Canned Tuna	__ Yellow and Red Onion
__ Vanilla Extract	__ Mayonnaise	__ Spinach
__ Allspice	__ Olive Oil	__ Butternut Squash
__ Sea Salt	__ Coconut Oil	__ Rosemary
__ NuNatural Stevia	__ Dijon Mustard	__ Avocado
__ Balsamic Vinegar	__ Clarified Butter	__ Lime and Lemon
__ Dried Oregano	__ Almond Flour (Whole Foods, Mothers Market, Sprouts)	__ Fresh Cilantro
__ Dill	__ Coconut Flour (Whole Foods, Mothers Market, Sprouts)	__ Tomatoes
__ Ground Cumin	__ Almond butter	__ Cauliflower
__ Ground Cayenne Pepper		__ Carrots

__ Dried Thyme

__ Dried Basil

__ Paprika

DRIED INGREDIENTS

__ Walnuts

__ Pecans

__ Ground Flaxseed

__ Pumpkin Seeds

MEATS

__ Farm-Fresh Eggs

__ Prosciutto

__ Chorizo

__ Chicken Breast

__ Bacon (Turkey Bacon)

__ Beef Tri-Tip

__ Mahimahi (Or Salmon)

__ Pork

__ Ground Turkey

__ Lean Ground Beef

__ Pork Chops

__ Ground chicken

__ Garlic Cloves

__ Celery Sticks

__ Green Chilies

__ Green Onions

__ Jalapeno

__ Romaine

__ Asparagus

__ Radish

__ Spaghetti Squash

__ Broccoli

__ Zucchini

WEEK EIGHT

	Breakfast	Lunch	Dinner
Monday	Chicken Chorizo "No-Potato" Hash	Beef Stew	Grilled Salmon with Avocado Salsa
Tuesday	Tuna and Egg Sandwich	Cauliflower Tabbouleh	Grilled Chicken with Greek Sweet Potatoes
Wednesday	Dijon Egg and Veggie Scramble	Herb Turkey Burgers with Zucchini Buns	Simple Herb-Crusted Salmon
Thursday	Kitchen Hash	Tuna-Salad Celery Boats with Avocado and Dill	Hatch Chile Meatballs
Friday	Breakfast Zucchini Pancakes	Pork-Fried Cauliflower Rice	Roasted Garlic, Spinach, and Mushroom–Stuffed Pork Chops
Saturday	Breakfast Burrito	Zucchini Pesto Roll-Ups	Pork Burgers
Sunday	Granola Cereal	Pepper Poppers	Simple Bacon and Spinach–Stuffed Chicken

WEEK EIGHT GROCERY LIST

SEASONINGS	OTHERS	PRODUCE
__ Salt	__ Olive Oil	__ Red and Yellow Onion
__ Pepper	__ Canned Tuna	__ Cilantro
__ Vanilla	__ Almond Flour (Whole Foods, Mothers Market, Sprouts)	__ Zucchini
__ Sage	__ Dijon Mustard	__ Red Pepper
__ Ground Fennel	__ Honey	__ Bell Pepper
__ Garlic Powder	__ Almond Butter	__ Sweet Potatoes
__ Dried Oregano	__ Coconut Oil	__ Carrots
__ Red-Pepper Flakes	__ Beef Stock or Beef Broth	__ Green Peas
__ Ground Coriander	__ Dijon Mustard	__ Green Onion
__ Cumin	__ Coconut Flour (Whole Foods, Mothers Market, Sprouts)	__ Spinach
__ Paprika Powder	__ White-Wine Vinegar	__ Tomatoes and Cherry Tomatoes
__ Onion Powder		__ Avocado
__ Dried Thyme		__ Celery
		__ Rosemary
		__ Thyme
		__ Cauliflower

DRIED INGREDIENTS

__ Pecans

__ Almonds

__ Dried Cranberries

__ Shredded Coconut

__ Walnuts

MEATS

__ Chorizo

__ Chicken Breast

__ Eggs

__ Ham

__ Beef Tri-Tip

__ Ground Pork

__ Ground Turkey

__ Italian Sausage

__ Salmon

__ Pork Chops

__ Ground Chicken

__ Bacon (Turkey)

__ Parsley

__ Mint

__ Lemon and Lime

__ Garlic

__ Oregano

__ Basil

__ Baby Sweet Peppers

__ Kale

__ Arugula

__ Portobello Button
   Mushrooms

WEEK NINE

	Breakfast	Lunch	Dinner
Monday	Brussels Sprout and Spinach Truffle Frittata	Spicy Redfish Stew	Zucchini and Ground Beef
Tuesday	Easy Breakfast Scramble	Lemon and Almond Cauliflower Rice	Chicken Piccata
Wednesday	Roasted Eggplant Stacks	Chicken Fajita Salad	Grilled Salmon with Avocado Salsa
Thursday	Porridge with Berries	Creamy Zucchini Pasta with Shrimp	Zucchini Fettuccine Alfredo
Friday	Salmon and Zucchini Fritters	Vegetable Cauliflower Rice	Simple Herb-Crusted Salmon
Saturday	Scrambled Eggs with Mushrooms and Pine Nuts	Grain-Free Salmon Rolls	Pork Burgers
Sunday	Asparagus and Basil Omelets	Fajitas	Crispy Skin Salmon

WEEK NINE GROCERY LIST

SEASONINGS	OTHERS	PRODUCE
__ Garlic Powder	__ Truffle Oil	__ Brussels Sprouts
__ Paprika	__ Clarified Butter	__ Fresh Spinach
__ Salt	__ Jarred Sundried Tomatoes	__ Garlic Cloves
__ Pepper	__ Olive Oil	__ Avocado
__ Herbes de Provence	__ Balsamic Vinegar	__ Parsley
__ Sea Salt	__ Coconut Oil	__ Sweet Potatoes
__ Red-Pepper Flakes	__ Almond Flour (Whole Foods, Mothers Market, Sprouts)	__ Yellow and Red Onions
__ Cumin	__ Capers	__ Bell Pepper
__ Oregano	__ Chicken Stock (Broth)	__ Mushrooms
	__ Coconut Cream	__ Eggplant
	__ Coconut Water	__ Tomatoes
		__ Berries
		__ Zucchini
		__ Dill

DRIED INGREDIENTS	MEATS	__ Asparagus
		__ Basil
__ Shredded, Unsweetened Coconut	__ Ground Beef	__ Sage
__ Raw Walnuts	__ Eggs	__ Chives
__ Sliced Almonds	__ Smoked Salmon	__ Cilantro

__ Raw Pepitas (Shelled Pumpkin Seeds)

__ Ground Flaxseed

__ Whole Almonds

__ Sausage

__ Choice of Fish

__ Chicken Breast

__ Shrimp

__ Salmon Fillet (Skin On)

__ Lemon and Lime

__ Cauliflower

__ Red-Leaf or Romaine Lettuce

__ Tomatoes

__ Avocado

__ Large Cucumber

__ One Peach

__ One Small Mango

__ Jalapeno

__ Celery

WEEK TEN

	Breakfast	Lunch	Dinner
Monday	Baked Eggs in Prosciutto-Filled Portobello Mushroom Caps	Beef and Butternut Squash Stew with Rosemary and Balsamic Vinegar	Chicken Broccoli Alfredo
Tuesday	Scrambled Eggs with Basil and Walnuts	Fish Tacos	Lemon, Garlic, and Herb Pork Chops
Wednesday	No-Oat Oatmeal	Pork-Fried Cauliflower Rice	Zucchini and Ground Beef
Thursday	Kitchen Hash	Tuna-Salad Celery Boats with Avocado and Dill	Hatch Chile Meatballs
Friday	Grilled Garlic Mushrooms with Bacon	Turkey Lettuce-Wrap Tacos with Chilies, Cumin, Cilantro, Lime and Tomato-Avocado Salsa	Herb Spinach Chicken Burgers
Saturday	Zucchini Pancake Breakfast Tower	Vegetable Cauliflower Rice	Simple Bacon and Spinach–Stuffed Chicken
Sunday	Pumpkin Porridge	Ground-Beef Skillet	Easy Chicken Dinner in 1...2...3

WEEK TEN GROCERY LIST

SEASONINGS	OTHERS	PRODUCE
		__ Medium to Large Portobello Mushroom
__ Black Pepper	__ Almond Milk (Unsweetened)	__ Parsley
__ Salt	__ Coconut Milk	__ Thyme
__ Ground Cinnamon	__ Pumpkin Puree	__ Fresh Basil
__ Ground Nutmeg	__ Diced, Jarred Roasted Red Pepper	__ Banana
__ Ground Ginger	__ Low-Sodium Beef Broth or Beef Stock	__ Fresh Berries
__ Garlic Powder	__ Coconut Amino	__ Yellow and Red Bell Peppers
__ Onion Powder	__ Canned Tuna	__ Yellow and Red Onion
__ Vanilla Extract	__ Mayonnaise	__ Spinach
__ Allspice	__ Olive Oil	__ Butternut Squash
__ Sea Salt	__ Coconut Oil	__ Rosemary
__ Nunatural Stevia	__ Dijon Mustard	__ Avocado
__ Balsamic Vinegar	__ Clarified Butter	__ Lime and Lemon
__ Dried Oregano	__ Almond Flour (Whole Foods, Mothers Market, Sprouts)	__ Fresh Cilantro
__ Dill	__ Coconut Flour (Whole Foods, Mothers Market, Sprouts)	__ Tomatoes
__ Ground Cumin	__ Almond Butter	__ Cauliflower
__ Ground Cayenne Pepper		__ Carrots

__ Dried Thyme

__ Dried Basil

__ Paprika

MEATS

__ Farm-Fresh Eggs

__ Prosciutto

__ Chorizo

DRIED INGREDIENTS

__ Chicken Breast

__ Walnuts

__ Bacon (Turkey)

__ Pecans

__ Beef Tri-Tip

__ Ground Flaxseed

__ Mahimahi (or Salmon)

__ Pumpkin Seeds

__ Pork

__ Ground Turkey

__ Lean Ground Beef

__ Pork Chops

__ Ground Chicken

__ Garlic Cloves

__ Celery Sticks

__ Green Chilies

__ Green Onions

__ Jalapeno

__ Romaine

__ Asparagus

__ Radish

__ Spaghetti Squash

__ Broccoli

__ Zucchini

PART THREE

RECIPES

BREAKFAST

Baked Eggs in Portobello Mushroom Caps

Did you know that you can bake eggs in a portobello mushroom cap? Well, you can. It's a little challenging because, depending on the shape of the cap, you might experience the mishap of an escaping egg. They can slide off the mushroom if you aren't careful. Here's how I did it.

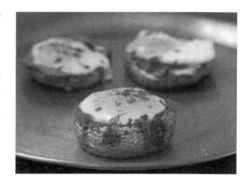

Ingredients
- farm-fresh eggs
- portobello mushroom caps (medium to large)
- sliced prosciutto
- black pepper
- fresh parsley or thyme
- a little olive oil

Instructions
1. Clean the portobello mushroom caps with a damp cloth. Remove the stem, and scrape out the gills so that you have a well deep enough for the egg.
2. Rub a little bit of olive oil on the outside of the mushroom to help it cook and keep it from sticking to the pan. Arrange the caps on a baking sheet.
3. Place one slice of prosciutto inside the mushroom cap.
4. Crack each egg into a small bowl, and then carefully slide it into a prosciutto-filled mushroom cap.

5. Sprinkle these with black pepper and fresh herbs of choice (I used parsley, but thyme would be great as well). The prosciutto is salty, so I don't recommend adding salt.

6. *Very carefully* place the baking pan into the oven (preheated to 375 degrees Fahrenheit), and bake for twenty to thirty minutes. The amount of time required depends on how thick your mushrooms are and how well done you like your eggs.

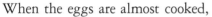 Scrambled Eggs with Basil and Walnut

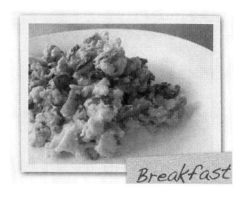

Breakfast

Ingredients
3 eggs
1/2 cup fresh basil, chopped
1/3 cup walnuts, chopped
salt and pepper

Instructions
Whisk the eggs in a bowl, and then place them in a frying pan on medium heat, stirring constantly. When the eggs are almost cooked, add the basil and continue cooking for one minute or until the eggs are fully cooked.

Add salt and pepper to taste.

Remove from heat, and stir in the walnuts before serving.

🌿 No-Oat Oatmeal

Ingredients

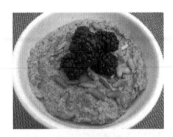

- 1 small handful walnuts
- 1 small handful pecans
- 2 tablespoons ground flaxseed
- 1/2 to 1 teaspoon ground cinnamon
- 1 pinch ground nutmeg
- 1 pinch ground ginger
- 1 tablespoon almond butter
- 1 banana, mashed
- 3 eggs

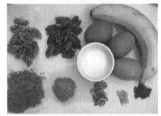

- 1/4 cup unsweetened almond milk (add more if you prefer it a little runny)
- 2 teaspoons pumpkin seeds
- 1 handful goji or other fresh berries

Instructions

Add walnuts, pecans, flaxseed and spices to a food processor, and pulse it down to a coarse grain, making sure to stop before it's totally ground into a powder. Set this aside.

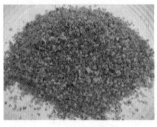

Whisk together eggs and almond milk (or use a blender) until the consistency thickens to resemble a loose custard. Thoroughly blend together the mashed banana and almond butter, and add it to the custard, mixing well.

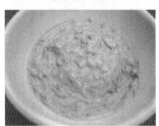

Stir in the nut mixture. Microwave or gently warm on the stove until it reaches your desired consistency; this should only take a few minutes. In both cases, stir the mixture frequently as it cooks.

Sprinkle pumpkin seeds and berries on top. Add more almond milk if you want.

Kitchen Hash

Ingredients

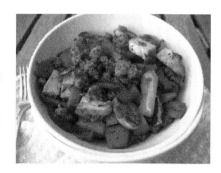

- 1pound chorizo
- 1/2 pound leftover chicken, diced
- 1 yellow bell pepper, diced and seeds removed
- 1 mild green chili pepper, diced and seeds removed
- 1/2 yellow onion, diced
- 1 sweet potato or yam, diced
- 1 package of button mushrooms, sliced
- sprinkle of garlic powder and onion powder
- pinch of salt and pepper

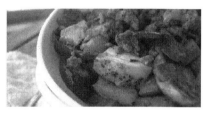

Instructions

1. Add chorizo to a large skillet over medium heat.
2. Use a spatula to break up your chorizo, and cook it until it's completely cooked through.
3. Use a slotted spoon to place the cooked chorizo to sit in a bowl while you cook the rest of your meal.
4. Place onions and sweet potatoes in your leftover chorizo grease and seasonings. Stir, and cover to cook down and steam, stirring randomly.
5. Once your sweet potatoes begin to soften, add your yellow bell pepper and green chili pepper, and stir to let cook down. After about four to five minutes, add your mushrooms.
6. Once the mushrooms are soft, add your cooked leftover chicken and chorizo back to the mix, and add your seasonings and salt and pepper (you won't need much because of the chorizo seasonings leftover in your pan).
7. Keep stirring your hash around until the sweet potatoes are cooked to your liking and flavors are completely incorporated.
8. Top with avocado and eat up.

◼Grilled Garlic Mushrooms with Bacon

Ingredients
2 cups mushrooms, sliced
3 slices of bacon, diced
3 tablespoons parsley, finely chopped
3 tablespoons olive oil
3 garlic cloves, finely chopped
salt and pepper

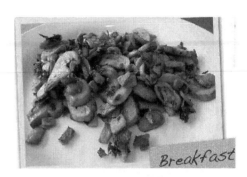
Breakfast

Instructions
Preheat the grill on medium-high heat.
Place all ingredients in a bowl, and combine well.
Place the ingredients on the grill to cook, stirring occasionally for five to eight minutes or until the bacon has become slightly crispy and the mushrooms have begun to shrivel.
Add salt and pepper to taste. Serve immediately.

▪Zucchini Pancake Breakfast Tower

Ingredients (Pancakes)
- 1 zucchini
- 1 egg
- 2 tablespoons almond flour

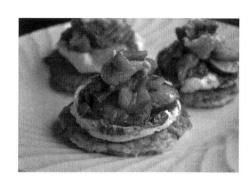

Ingredients (Tower)
- 2 eggs
- 1/2 cup fresh spinach
- 2 ounces turkey kielbasa
- 2 tablespoons guacamole
- 2 tablespoons diced, jarred roasted red pepper

Instructions

Shred the zucchini, and squeeze out all the water. Mix this with the egg and almond flour. Add salt and pepper to taste. Using a nonstick skillet, make the mixture into three pancakes. Go low and slow so that the inside cooks before the outside burns, about three minutes on each side. Set aside.

In three, 4-ounce ramekins (small ceramic or glass serving bowls), divide the spinach, egg, and turkey kielbasa in each ramekin, and microwave for one minute.

To assemble, place one zucchini pancake on the bottom, add the egg-spinach-kielbasa layer on top of that, and then add guacamole and diced red peppers over the top.

🌿 Pumpkin Porridge

Ingredients

- 3 eggs
- 2 tablespoons coconut milk
- 1/3 cup and 2 tablespoons pumpkin puree
- 1/4 teaspoon vanilla extract
- 1 tablespoon coconut oil
- allspice
- pinch of Celtic sea salt
- 20 to 30 drops NuNaturals liquid stevia
- chopped walnuts

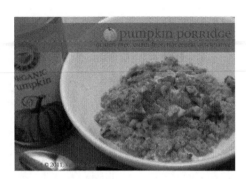

Instructions

1. In a mixing bowl, whisk the eggs.
2. To eggs, add 1/3 cup pumpkin puree, 1 tablespoon coconut milk, vanilla extract, a couple shakes of allspice, sea salt, and the stevia. Whisk together until smooth.
3. In a small saucepan on medium-high heat, melt the coconut oil.
4. Add the egg mixture to the saucepan, and whisk constantly until mixture resembles cottage cheese. This takes less than two or three minutes.
5. Remove from the heat quickly, and spoon into a bowl.
6. Top with 1 tablespoon of cream or coconut milk, 2 tablespoons of pumpkin, another shake of allspice, and chopped walnuts.

Chicken Chorizo "No Potato" Hash

Ingredients

1/2 red onion, chopped
1/2 chopped cilantro
4 large zucchini cut into 1/3-inch cubes
1 red pepper, seeded and chopped
6 to 8 ounces Mexican chorizo
2 cups cooked chicken, chopped or shredded
1 tablespoon oil, if needed
salt and pepper

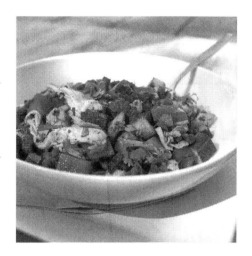

Instructions

Heat a large skillet over medium-high heat. Brown the chorizo for two to three minutes, and then add the chicken until warmed through. Remove the chorizo and chicken, and set this aside.

Add the onions to the skillet, and sauté for one minute. Add the zucchini, red pepper, and a tablespoon of oil if needed. Sauté for two to three minutes until just cooked but not mushy. Salt and pepper to taste. Then add the protein back in.

Remove from the heat, and stir in the cilantro. Serve immediately.

(This is a *great* recipe to make use of leftover chicken or a store-bought rotisserie chicken.)

Tuna and Egg Sandwich

Ingredients

1 bell pepper cut in half
1 195-gram can of tuna
1 egg
salt

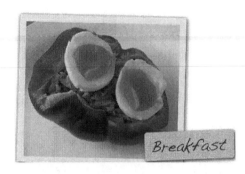

Instructions

Boil the egg for five to six minutes
or until desired firmness has been
reached. Cool the egg, and then peel it and cut it in half.
Place the tuna on the bottom of the bell pepper half, and place the egg halves
on top. Add salt if desired before serving.

Dijon Egg and Veggie Scramble

Ingredients

- 1 egg
- 2 egg whites
- 1/2 red bell pepper
- 1/2 zucchini
- 1 large green onion
- 1/2 teaspoon salt
- 1/2 teaspoon each (use some or all) chili powder, coriander, cumin, paprika, turmeric, pepper, cayenne, or curry
- 2 tablespoons Dijon mustard
- 1 cup spinach
- sprinkle of raw goat cheese, optional but delicious

Instructions

In a large skillet, heat 1 tablespoon of olive or coconut oil. Add the bell pepper and zucchini, stirring frequently. Cook on medium-high heat until the zucchini becomes soft and slightly translucent (about three to five minutes).

Crack the eggs, and add the whole egg and egg whites to the zucchini-and-pepper mixture. Scramble as desired. While the eggs are still cooking, add green onion, salt, and spices.

Continue to cook the eggs until they become fluffy and solid. Remove from the heat, and toss with Dijon mustard, spinach, and goat cheese.

Serve, and enjoy immediately.

Breakfast Zucchini Pancakes

Ingredients
- 1 zucchini of medium size
- 1 large egg
- 1 green onion of medium size
- 2 1/2 tablespoons of olive oil

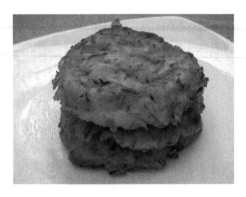

Instructions
Grate the zucchini into a bowl, chop the green onion, and mix both together. Add one large egg to the mixture, and mix thoroughly, adding salt and pepper. Put three mounds of zucchini mixture into the pan, and fry it by pressing down until lightly browned, and then turn it to brown the other side.

Now you have some amazing breakfast pancakes.

🖤Breakfast Burrito

Ingredients

- sliced ham (one that is large enough to fold and of medium thickness so that it doesn't break when wrapped—possibly more than one slice)
- 2 eggs (or egg whites)
- 1/4 cup chopped veggies (spinach, black olives, bell pepper, tomato, etc.)
- salsa, guacamole, and cilantro (optional)

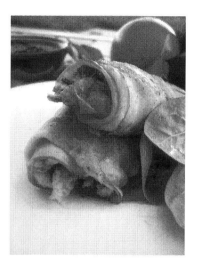

Instructions

1. Sauté the veggies in a small bit of oil over medium to high heat.
2. In a small bowl, whisk the eggs, and poor the veggie mix in.
3. Using a spatula, scramble the mix until cooked through. Take the eggs out of the pan.
4. Roll the ham around the eggs, and place back onto the skillet. Grill for a few seconds on each side until the ham is slightly brown.
5. Serve with salsa, guacamole, and a sprig of fresh cilantro on top.

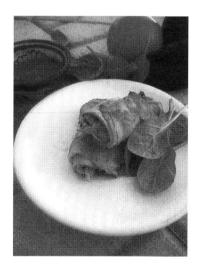

Granola Cereal

Ingredients

1 cup pecans
1 cup almonds
1 tablespoon honey
2 tablespoons almond butter
3 tablespoons almond butter
3 tablespoons coconut oil
1/2 teaspoon vanilla
1 pinch salt
1/2 cup dried cranberries
1/2 cup shredded coconut

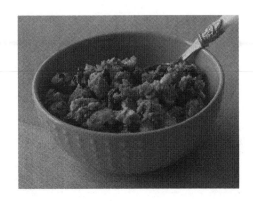

Instructions

Place the almonds and pecans (or any other nuts of your choosing) in a food processor and pulse a few times (but not too much). In a medium saucepan, melt the coconut oil (or butter), and whisk in the honey, vanilla, salt, and almond butter. Pour this mixture into the food processor with your nuts, and pulse a few more times to combine. Add cranberries (or dried fruit of your choosing) and shredded coconut, and pulse one last time. Spread the mixture out on a parchment-lined baking sheet, and bake at 365 degrees Fahrenheit for twenty to thirty minutes.

You can eat this dry, covered with coconut or almond milk (like cereal), or as a topper for fresh fruit.

◢ ▪ Brussels Sprouts and Spinach Truffle Frittata

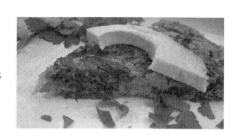

Ingredients
- 8 eggs, whisked
- 2 cups Brussels sprouts, cut in fourths
- 5 to 6 cups fresh spinach
- 3 tablespoons clarified butter.
- 2 teaspoons truffle oil
- 2 garlic cloves, minced
- 1 teaspoon garlic powder
- 1/2 teaspoon paprika
- salt and pepper to taste
- avocado to garnish
- chopped parsley to garnish

Instructions
1. Preheat the oven to 375 degrees Fahrenheit.
2. Place a large skillet over medium to high heat, and add the ghee. Once the pan is hot, add the minced garlic, Brussels sprouts, and a bit of salt and pepper. Let this cook until browned on one side, and then use a spatula or flip of the wrist to move the sprouts around.
3. After about five to six minutes, add the spinach, covering it so that it will steam and cook. Cook it for about three to four more minutes, until the spinach is cooked down and soft.
4. While spinach is finishing cooking, whisk your eggs in a large bowl, and then add the truffle oil, garlic powder, paprika, salt, and pepper, along with the cooked spinach and Brussels sprouts. Mix well.
5. Pour into a cast-iron skillet.
6. Place this in the oven, and cook for fifteen to eighteen minutes, depending on the size of the skillet. When you press on the middle, and it pushes back a bit, you'll know the frittata is done cooking.
7. Top the frittata with a dribble of truffle oil, avocado, and parsley.

Easy Breakfast Scramble

Ingredients
- 1 sweet potato, diced
- 1/2 yellow onion, diced
- 1 mild green chili pepper, sliced
- 1 container of sliced mushrooms (about 6 to 8 ounces)
- 1/2 pound grass-fed beef
- 5 eggs
- 1 garlic clove, minced
- 1 tablespoon ghee
- 1 tablespoon herbes de Provence
- salt and pepper to taste

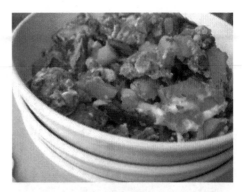

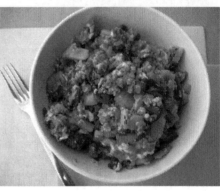

Instructions
1. Slice and dice everything so that it's ready to go.
2. Place a large skillet over medium heat, and add the ghee and minced garlic to the pan.
3. When the garlic becomes fragrant, add your sweet potatoes, yellow onion, poblano pepper, and mushrooms. Cover, and let cook for around three minutes.
4. Add your beef, breaking it up with a wooden spoon or spatula. Cover, and let the meat cook through (about three to five minutes).
5. Once the beef is almost cooked through, crack yours eggs directly into the pan, and add your herbes de Provence, salt, and pepper.
6. Use your spoon to break up the eggs and help them cook through, as well as to incorporate all the seasonings.
7. Once the eggs are cooked through, taste it to make sure there is enough salt and seasonings, and add more if needed.
8. Then serve.

❤Roasted Eggplant Stacks

Ingredients

1 Italian eggplant cut into 1/2-inch rounds

1 tomato, sliced into 1/4-inch rounds

fresh ground pork sausage or other ground meat of your choice formed into patties about the same size as your eggplant rounds

poached eggs

finely diced sundried tomatoes

minced parsley

extra-virgin olive oil

balsamic vinegar

coconut oil

sea salt

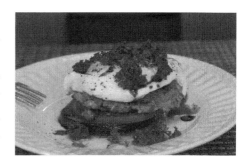

Instructions

1. Brush both sides of your eggplant rounds with coconut oil, and sprinkle them with sea salt.
2. Broil the eggplant rounds under you broiler on high heat for four to five minutes on one side, flip, and broil for three to four minutes on the other side or until they are tender and start to brown.
3. In the meantime, panfry your sausage patties until they are done all the way through.
4. Poach some eggs, slice the tomatoes, dice the sun-dried tomatoes, and mince the parsley.
5. Now stack. Place a roasted eggplant round on a plate, top it with a tomato slice, a sausage patty, some diced sun-dried tomatoes, and a little bit of parsley.
6. Finish it all with a drizzle of olive oil, balsamic vinegar, and black pepper to taste.

🌿 Porridge with Berries

Ingredients

- 1/4 cup shredded, unsweetened coconut
- 1/4 cup raw walnuts
- 1/4 cup sliced almonds
- 2 tablespoons raw pepitas (shelled pumpkin seeds)
- 1 tablespoon flaxseed meal
- 1/2 cup hot water
- 1/2 cup berries (your choice or mixed)

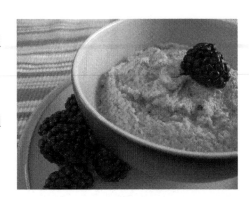

Instructions

1. Process coconut, walnuts, almonds, pepitas, and flaxseed together in a blender or food processor until finely ground and blade starts to seize.
2. Boil water in a kettle or in the microwave, and mix in honey if desired.
3. Stir the ground nuts into the hot water.
4. Heat in the microwave on high for thirty seconds. Stir once more. Let it sit for three to five minutes to thicken. Top off with berries of your choice. Enjoy.

Salmon and Zucchini Fritters

Ingredients

2 eggs
1 1/2 cup almond meal
100 grams smoked salmon, thinly sliced
2 large zucchini, roughly grated, liquid squeezed out
1 tablespoon chopped dill
salt and pepper
olive oil

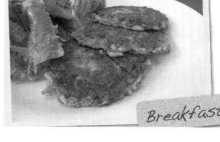

Instructions

Combine the eggs and almond meal in a bowl, and whisk until smooth. Stir in the smoked salmon, zucchini, dill salt, and pepper.

Place the oil in a frying pan over medium heat.

Scoop 1 tablespoonful of the smoked-salmon mixture into the pan, allowing room for spreading. Fry for two to three minutes on each side until golden and cooked through. Drain the fritter on absorbent paper.

Repeat with the remaining smoked-salmon mixture, adding oil to the pan between each batch as required. Serve with a simple green salad.

Scrambled Eggs with Mushroom and Pine Nuts

Ingredients

3 eggs
2 teaspoons onion, finely chopped
2 tablespoons chives, finely chopped
1 cup sliced mushrooms
1 tablespoon oil
1 tablespoon pine nuts
salt and pepper

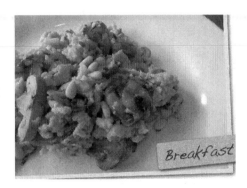

Breakfast

Instructions

Place the oil in a frying pan on medium heat, and fry the onions for three to four minutes until lightly browned. Remove the mushrooms from the pan. Whisk the eggs in a bowl, and then pour into the frying pan. Cook while stirring constantly.

When the eggs are almost cooked, add the chives, and continue cooking for one more minute or until the eggs are done.

Add salt and pepper to taste.

Remove from the heat, and stir in the mushrooms before serving.

Asparagus and Basil Omelet

Ingredients
5 asparagus stalks cut into 2.5 centimeter pieces
1 large clove garlic, finely chopped
1tablespoon oil
2/3 cup mushrooms, diced
4 eggs, beaten
1/2 cup fresh basil, roughly chopped
salt and pepper

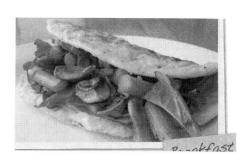

Instructions
Boil asparagus pieces for two to four minutes or until tender. Drain and set the asparagus aside.

Fry the garlic in oil for one minute. Add the mushrooms, and cook for two more minutes. Remove this from the pan, and mix with asparagus, chopped basil, salt, and pepper.

Heat up a frying pan lined with baking paper. Pour the beaten eggs onto the baking paper. When the bottom of the eggs has set, turn the mixture over by placing another sheet of baking paper on top and flipping the eggs onto it. Transfer this back to the heated frying pan, and cook it for an extra two to three minutes or until browned on the bottom.

To serve it, place the omelet on a plate, spoon the asparagus mixture onto one half, and then fold the omelet.

LUNCH

Beef and Butternut Squash Stew with Rosemary and Balsamic Vinegar

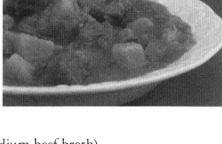

Ingredients

1 medium onion, diced

2 teaspoons olive oil (or more, depends on your pan)

1 pound beef tri-tip or top sirloin, cut in 1 1/2-inch cubes

3 cups butternut squash cubes, cut into 1 1/2-inch pieces

1 1/2 cups beef stock (or 1 can low-sodium beef broth)

1/4 cup water

1 tablespoon chopped fresh or frozen rosemary or 2 teaspoons finely chopped dried rosemary (or more if you really like rosemary)

2 tablespoons balsamic vinegar (or more, depending on taste)

salt and freshly ground black pepper to taste

Instructions

Put one teaspoon of olive oil into a pan, heat it for a minute, and then sauté the onions until they soften and are just starting to brown. Remove the onions from the pan, add a second teaspoon of olive oil and the beef cubes, and sauté this until the beef is well browned on all sides (about five minutes). Pour in 1/4 cup water, and scrape up any browned bits from the bottom of the pan. Then add sautéed onions, 2 cups of squash cubes, rosemary, balsamic vinegar, and beef stock. Lower the heat, cover the pan, and cook at a gentle simmer until squash dissolves into the liquid. (Depending on how well your pan lid fits, you may need to add a little water at this point.)

Cut the remaining cup of squash cubes in half again to make smaller pieces, and add them to the stew. Taste for seasoning to see if you want to add a tiny bit more balsamic vinegar. Cook for twenty minutes more or until squash is cooked through. Season with salt and freshly ground black pepper, and serve it hot.

Fish Tacos

Ingredients

- 1 pound mahimahi (or whatever is local, wild, and fresh)
- 1 teaspoon dried oregano
- 1 teaspoon garlic powder
- 2 tablespoons extra-virgin olive oil
- 1 small head green cabbage or romaine lettuce (four large leaves reserved; the rest shredded)
- 1 medium ripe avocado, sliced
- 1 small lime
- 2 tablespoons fresh cilantro, chopped
- 1 large ripe tomato, chopped

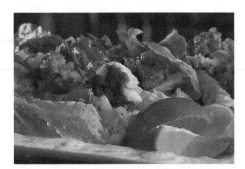

Instructions

1. Pat the fish dry with a paper towel. Combine the oregano and garlic powder. Heat the oven to broil.
2. Press the oregano mixture into the fish. Place the fish on a wire rack under the broiler for ten minutes, turning over after five minutes.
3. Make sure the internal temperature is 150 degrees Fahrenheit, and then remove it from the oven, and tent it with foil.
4. Let it rest for five to ten minutes while you steam your favorite green veggies.
5. Divide the fish into four portions (two per person). Place each in one of the four cabbage leaves.
6. Top with shredded cabbage, avocado, lime juice, cilantro, and tomato.

Pork-Fried Cauliflower Rice

Ingredients

- 1 tablespoon olive oil
- 1 head cauliflower, chopped and blended in the food processor to a rice-like consistency
- 1 cup pork, cooked and chopped
- 2 carrots, peeled and diced
- 1/2 onion, chopped
- 2 cloves garlic, minced
- 1/4 cup coconut aminos
- (soy sauce equivalent)
- 2 eggs
- salt and pepper

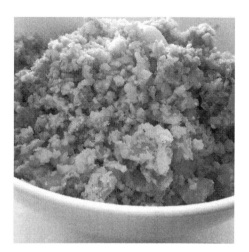

Instructions

1. When you have all of the above ingredients prepared, heat the olive oil in a pan over medium heat, add the onions, carrots, and garlic, and cook until they start to become soft. Add the blended cauliflower, and cook thoroughly.
2. Next, add the pork and coconut aminos, and continue to sauté.
3. In a bowl, crack the eggs, and then whisk them. Add this to the pan, stirring for a few minutes until they are cooked.
4. Season with salt and pepper to taste

Tuna-Salad Celery Boats with Avocado and Dill

Ingredients

- 1 can tuna
- 1 to 2 tablespoons paleo mayo
- 2 tablespoons red onion, diced finely
- 1/2 an avocado, cut into 1/2-inch cubes
- 5 to 6 cherry tomatoes, halved
- 1/2 teaspoon (or more) garlic
- 1 teaspoon dill
- 1/2 teaspoon lemon juice
- 5 to 6 celery sticks

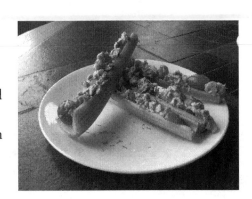

Instructions

1. I would strongly advise you to pay attention to the celery you buy. I've had those gigantic sticks before, and they would work best for this method. However, as you can see in the pictures, the small ones will do—it's just trickier getting them to hold the salad.
2. Mix the tuna with the mayonnaise, garlic, dill, lemon juice, and onion.
3. Add the avocado and onion, and stir. (Not too much! You want the avocado to remain intact! Or maybe you don't...it's up to you.)
4. Spoon the mixture into your celery sticks, or you can use these in lettuce wraps or as a salad topper with spinach...the possibilities are endless.

Turkey Lettuce-Wrap Tacos with Chilies, Cumin, Cilantro, Lime and Tomato-Avocado Salsa

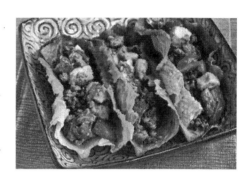

Ingredients

1 tablespoon olive oil

1 teaspoon minced garlic

1 to 2 tablespoons diced green chilies

1 teaspoon ground cumin

1/4 teaspoon ground cayenne pepper

1 1/2 pounds ground turkey

1/2 teaspoon salt

1/2 cup thinly sliced green onions

1 large bunch cilantro, finely chopped (about 1 cup in tacos and 1/4 cup in salsa)

2 tablespoons fresh lime juice

2 large heads romaine lettuce

2 medium avocados, diced

1 1/2 cups finely chopped cherry tomatoes

1/4 cup finely chopped cilantro

2 tablepsoons fresh lime juice

2 tablepsoons olive oil (optional)

sea salt to taste

Instructions

Heat the olive oil in a heavy frying pan, add minced garlic and diced green chilies, and sauté for about one minute. (I use a nonstick pan. If you use fresh garlic and chilies, they may have to cook a bit longer.) Add cumin and ground chipotle or cayenne, and cook for one minute more. Then add the turkey and salt, and cook this over medium-high heat, breaking it apart as it cooks. Cook for about five minutes, or until the turkey starts to brown.

While the turkey cooks, thinly slice the green onions and set them aside. Wash the cilantro, spin it dry or dry it with paper towels, and finely chop it. Cut off the root end of the lettuce, discard the tough outer leaves, and wash and then dry in a salad spinner or with paper towels.

When the turkey is lightly browned, add sliced green onions and cook for about two minutes. Turn off the heat, and stir in 1 cup of chopped cilantro and 2 tablespoons of lime juice.

To make the salsa, peel and dice the avocados. Place them in a glass or plastic bowl, and toss with lime juice. Stir in the chopped tomatoes, chopped cilantro, and olive oil, and then season to taste with salt.

To assemble tacos, put two to three large spoonfuls of turkey mixture into each piece of lettuce. (I used the inner, more folded pieces of lettuce and saved the flatter outer pieces for a salad.) Top this with salsa.

✿ ❤ Vegetable Cauliflower Rice

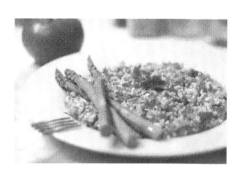

Ingredients
- 1/2 small organic red onion
- 2 organic garlic cloves
- 1/2 organic white cauliflower bunch
- 6 to 12 organic asparagus shoots (depending on how many you want)
- 1 to 2 large organic carrot
- 1 to 2 organic celery stalk
- 1 bunch of organic Italian parsley
- 1 bunch of organic cilantro
- 1 large organic tomato
- 1 to 2 tablespoons organic virgin coconut oil (for frying)
- sea salt
- organic black peppercorn

Instructions
1. Chop the onions and garlic, and let this sit for ten minutes.
2. Chop (pulse) the cauliflower in a food processor, until it is the size of short rice grains. Add the cauliflower rice to a large mixing bowl, and set aside.
3. Add salt to the asparagus, and steam it until tender. Set aside.
4. Chop the carrots and celery into chunks, and then chop (pulse) the carrots, celery, and herbs in a food processor. Add this to the mixing bowl. Set aside.
5. Dice the tomato, and then add to mixing bowl.
6. In a small frying pan, on medium-low heat, lightly fry the onions and garlic for about three to five minutes. (If you can tolerate the strength of raw onion and garlic, you can skip this step and just add them to the mixing bowl.)
7. Once the onions are softened, remove them from the heat. Set them aside to cool.

8. Mix all the ingredients in the large mixing bowl.
9. Add the onions and garlic once cooled. Mix well.
10. Add salt and pepper. Check for flavor, and make necessary adjustments.
11. Once ready, distribute the rice mix onto two plates, and then top off with steamed asparagus.
12. Serve, and enjoy.

■Ground-Beef Skillet

Ingredients

1 pound ground beef
16 ounces radishes, quartered
5 ounces carrots, diced
3 cups spinach
3 tablespoons Dijon mustard
salt, pepper, and garlic powder to
taste

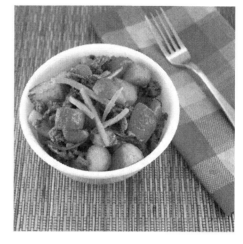

Instructions

Heat 1 to 2 tablespoons of oil in
a large skillet over medium-high
heat. Add the radishes and carrots,
and season them with salt, pepper, and garlic powder to taste. Sauté for five
to six minutes or until halfway tender. Push the veggies to the sides of the
pan, and add the ground beef in the middle. Cook the ground beef all the
way through. Drain the excess fat, and combine the meat with the veggies.
Add the spinach and Dijon mustard. Stir this, and cook it until the spinach
has wilted and the veggies are tender (cover the pan if necessary to soften the
veggies).

Beef Stew

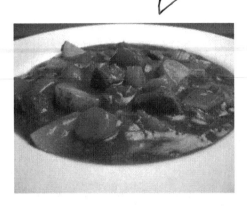

Ingredients

1 pound stewing beef
2 teaspoons coconut oil or olive oil
4 cups beef stock
1 cup onion, chopped
1 cup celery, chopped
3 carrots, peeled and chopped
1 diced tomato
1/2 teaspoon freshly chopped rosemary
1/2 teaspoon chopped thyme
sea salt and black pepper to taste

Instructions

In a large saucepan over medium-high heat, combine the onions, celery, carrots, and cooking oil. Cook for three to five minutes, stirring constantly.

Add the beef to the saucepan, followed by the tomato, beef stock, rosemary, and thyme. Season to taste with salt and pepper.

Cover the saucepan, and cook for about one hour, allowing the stew to simmer. Stir a few times during the cooking process.

Remove the lid, and cook uncovered for about forty-five minutes. If the mixture is too thick at the end of the cooking process, you can add a little bit of water or stock.

✐ ■ Cauliflower Tabbouleh

Ingredients

- 2 medium-size cauliflower heads
- 1 1/2 cups finely cut *(not chopped) fresh* flat-leaf parsley,
- 1/2 cup finely cut *(not chopped) fresh* mint
- 3 tomatoes, *diced*
- sea salt and crushed black pepper *to taste*
- 6 tablespoons extra-virgin olive oil
- 3 tablespoons lemon juice
- 2 cloves garlic, *minced*

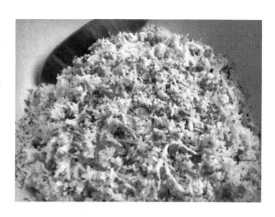

Instructions

Grate the cauliflower over the fine side of a grater. (*Note: A food processor with a grater-blade will make life a lot easier.*)

Pour the grated cauliflower into a large bowl, and carefully blend in the parsley, mint, and tomato with two large spoons.

Season with sea salt and crushed black pepper to taste.

Put the olive oil, lemon juice, and minced garlic in a shaker, and give it a few shakes.

Drizzle all the dressing over the salad, and give it a few tosses with the spoons.

Serve as a side, relax, and enjoy!

Herbed Turkey Burgers with Zucchini Buns

Ingredients

- 8 to 10 ounces ground, organic, lean turkey meat
- 2 tablespoons fresh oregano, chopped
- 2 garlic cloves, minced
- 4 thick slices of zucchini (or eggplant, summer squash, etc.)
- olive-oil spray
- salt and pepper to taste

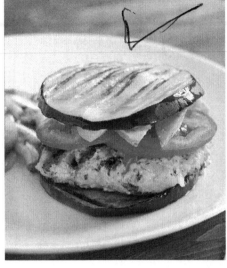

Instructions

1. In a large bowl, combine the turkey meat, oregano, and garlic cloves, and mix with your hands until fully combined. Form the mixture into two patties, and set it aside.
2. Heat a grill pan (or outdoor grill) to medium-high heat.
3. Spray the zucchini on both sides and sprinkle with salt and pepper.
4. Add the zucchini to the grill pan, and cook for two to three minutes per side, until you have nice grill marks and the zucchini still holds its shape.
5. Add the turkey burgers to the grill, cooking for three to five minutes per side, until cooked through.
6. Serve the burgers between the zucchini slices, and add your preferred toppings (sliced tomato, avocado, etc.).
7. Enjoy!

Pork-Fried Cauliflower Rice

Ingredients

- 1 tablespoon olive oil
- 1 head cauliflower, chopped and blended in the food processor to a rice-like consistency
- 1 cup pork, cooked and chopped
- 2 carrots, peeled and diced
- 1/2 onion, chopped
- 2 cloves garlic, minced
- 1/4 cup coconut aminos
- 2 eggs
- salt and pepper

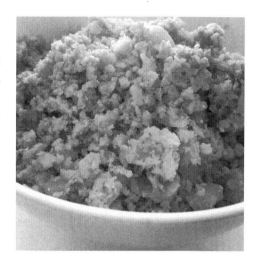

Instructions

1. When you have all of the above ingredients prepared, heat the olive oil in a pan over medium heat, and add the onions, carrots, and garlic, and cook them until they start to become soft.
2. Add the blended cauliflower, and cook it thoroughly.
3. Next, add the pork and coconut aminos, and continue to sauté everything.
4. In a bowl, crack the eggs, and then whisk them. Add the eggs to the pan, and stir for a few minutes until they are cooked.
5. Season with salt and pepper to taste.

Zucchini Pesto Roll-Ups

Ingredients

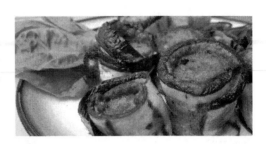

- 2 zucchinis, ends removed, sliced 1/4 inch thick lengthwise
- 4 Italian sausages (I use Boulder Sausage brand)
- 1/2 cup walnuts
- 1 cup fresh basil
- 1/3 cup olive oil
- juice of 1 lemon
- 1 garlic clove
- salt and pepper to taste
- pinch of garlic powder
- 3 extra tablespoons olive oil to cook the zucchini in

Instructions

1. Heat up your grill.
2. Slice your zucchini with a knife or a mandolin.
3. Place your zucchini in a bowl with 3 tablespoons of olive oil, salt and pepper, and a pinch of garlic powder, and then use your hands to mix it and coat the zucchini.
4. Place the Italian sausages on the grill, along with your zucchini.
5. While the zucchini and sausages are cooking, make the pesto: combine the walnuts, garlic clove, and basil in a food processor. Then begin to add the olive oil while the food processor is still running.
6. Add your lemon juice and salt and pepper. Taste to see if you need more basil, lemon, or salt and pepper. I think more lemon juice goes a long way.
7. After your zucchini have cooked for about four to five minutes and show grill marks, flip them. Be sure to keep an eye on them, because they will burn rather quickly.

8. Once your zucchini and sausage are completely cooked through, remove them to cool.
9. When your zucchini are cool to the touch, use a spoon to spread the pesto down the center of the zucchini strip, and cut off an inch of sausage.
10. Place the sausage in the middle of the zucchini so that the cut sides are facing toward the outer ridges of the zucchini. You'll figure it out.
11. Wrap the zucchini around the sausage, and use a toothpick to hold it in place.

■Pepper Poppers

Ingredients

24 baby sweet peppers with tops,
seeds and ribs removed
1/2 cup finely diced onion
1 pound Italian sausage
1 teaspoon garlic powder
1 teaspoon dried oregano
1/2 teaspoon salt
4 cups finely chopped kale
juice of 1/2 lemon
2 eggs lightly beaten

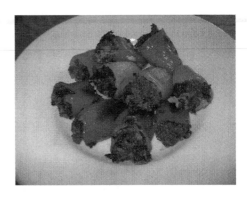

Instructions

In a large pan, sauté the sausage and onion in 2 tablespoons of oil until cooked through. Add the kale, salt, garlic powder, oregano, and lemon juice. Stir frequently until the kale is wilted, and then remove it from the heat. Prepare your peppers by slicing off the tops and paring out the seeds and ribs. Once the meat mixture is mostly cooled, add in the 2 eggs, and mix well. Stuff the peppers by packing them pretty tightly (using my hands worked best). Arrange them on a baking sheet.

Bake at 400 degrees Fahrenheit for fifteen minutes. Finish them under the broiler for one to two minutes or until brown on top.

Spicy Redfish Stew

Ingredients

1/2 cup finely chopped red onion or shallot

1 tablespoon olive oil

1 jar (12 ounces) roasted red bell peppers, drained and chopped

1 can (14 1/2 ounces) diced tomatoes with juice

1 teaspoon finely minced fresh garlic

1/4 teaspoon Red-pepper flakes (use more if you like it spicy)

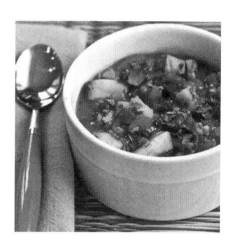

1/4 cup chopped fresh cilantro (plus more for garnish if desired)

1/2 teaspoon fresh lemon zest

2 teaspoons fresh lemon juice

8 to 10 ounces cod, halibut, or tilapia fillets cut into 1-inch pieces

salt and freshly ground black pepper to taste

Instructions

For best results with this recipe, use a small frying pan with high sides so that the fish pieces will be surrounded by liquid when you add them. I used an 8-inch pan.

Heat the olive oil in small frying pan, adding the chopped red onion or shallot. Sauté this over medium heat for about three to four minutes, until the onions are soft and starting to brown. Add chopped red bell peppers, diced tomatoes with juice, finely minced fresh garlic, and red-pepper flakes. Let the mixture simmer for ten minutes over medium-low heat until the garlic is cooked and flavors are well blended.

While the stew mixture simmers, zest and juice the lemon, and chop the cilantro. Cut the fish fillets into 1-inch pieces, and blot them dry with a paper towel if needed.

Add the lemon zest, lemon juice, and 1/4 cup chopped cilantro to stew mixture, add the fish pieces, and gently stir to combine. Let the stew simmer five to seven minutes or until the fish is barely turning opaque and some liquid from the fish is being released into the stew. Stir again, season to taste with salt and freshly ground black pepper, and serve it hot, with the additional chopped cilantro for garnish if desired.

✿ ◼ Lemon and Almond Cauliflower Rice

Ingredients

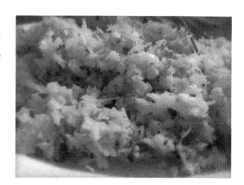

- 1 cauliflower head, *grated into a rice-like consistency over the coarse side of a grater*
- 3 1/2 ounces (100 grams) almonds, *roughly chopped*
- 1 lemon, *zested and juiced*
- crushed black pepper *to taste*
- 1 tablespoon coconut oil
- 2 tablespoons extra-virgin olive oil

Instructions

Heat the coconut oil in a large frying pan.

Add the riced cauliflower, and season it with a bit of crushed black pepper. Let it fry for five minutes or so while stirring occasionally.

Then add the lemon juice, stir it a bit, and keep frying for about another five minutes.

Add the chopped almonds and most of the lemon zest, stirring again to mix it all up, remove the pan from the heat, and drizzle the olive oil over it.

Give it one last stir before plating, and serve with the rest of the lemon zest sprinkled on top as garnish.

Chicken Fajita Salad

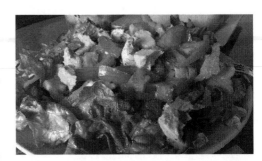

Ingredients
- 1 tablespoon coconut oil
- 1/2 yellow onion, diced
- 1/2 to 3/4 pound boneless, skinless chicken breasts
- 1/2 teaspoon ground cumin
- 2 teaspoons dried oregano
- 1/4 teaspoon sea salt (optional)
- 1 large bell pepper, chopped
- 1 large head red-leaf or romaine lettuce
- 2 medium tomatoes, diced
- 1 avocado

Instructions
1. Wash and chop the onion, bell pepper, and tomatoes.
2. Cut the chicken into 1/2-inch slices.
3. Heat a skillet over medium-high heat. When hot, add the coconut oil and onions. Sauté this until the onions are soft and slightly translucent.
4. Add the chicken, cumin, oregano, and sea salt to the onions, and continue to cook it, stirring often.
5. When the chicken has browned, add the peppers, cooking them until tender.
6. Meanwhile, wash and shred the lettuce. Divide the shredded lettuce between two plates.
7. Top the lettuce with the chicken-fajita mix, tomatoes, and sliced avocado.

Creamy Zucchini Pasta With Shrimp

Ingredients

- 4 zucchini, peeled and julienned
- 9 ounces shrimp
- 1 can diced tomatoes
- 1 avocado
- 1/4 cup fresh basil
- 2 tablespoons water
- salt and pepper

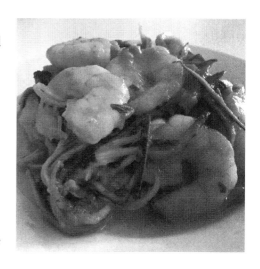

Instructions

1. In a pan, sauté the shrimp.
2. In a separate skillet, cook the zucchini.
3. In a food processor, blend the tomatoes, avocado, basil, water, salt, and pepper.
4. Once everything is done cooking, add the zucchini and sauce to the shrimp, and mix it until the sauce is heated.

Grain-Free Salmon Rolls

Ingredients

- 1 large cucumber
- 2 carrots
- 1 avocado
- 1 small cucumber
- 1 stalk of scallion
- 1 cup cooked salmon
- 1 fresh peach, skinned and sliced
- 1 small mango, skinned and sliced

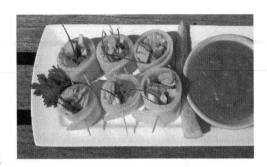

Instructions

1. Carefully set the mandolin for 1/8-inch thickness. Peel the cucumber, and set it in the mandolin.
2. Use the finger guard, please! Slice the cucumber on one side until you reach the seeds, and then turn it ninety degrees, and slice again. Keep turning until you have four sides sliced down to the seeds, which you can then discard. You should have eighteen to twenty slices if the cucumber was thick.
3. In the meantime, peel and cut the carrot into tiny slivers that will fit inside the large cucumber slice.
4. Open the avocado, and cut pieces that will fit inside the cucumber slice.
5. Peel and cut the small cucumber into slivers that will fit inside the large cucumber slice.
6. Cut the scallion and chunks of salmon into sizes that can fit right in.
7. Flatten out a large slice of cucumber on a flat working board, and start to fill it about a fourth of the way down.
8. Add a few slivers of carrot and cucumber, a chunk of avocado, strands of scallion, and a piece of salmon.

9. Roll the top edge over the filling, and tighten it, and then roll it up completely. If the cucumber is too long, you can cut off a few inches.
10. Pierce it with a toothpick to hold it all together.
11. To make the peach-mango sauce, puree the peach and mango slices in a mini processor. Serve the puree in a small dish next to the rolls and some lemon.

Fajitas

Ingredients

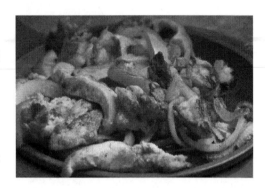

- 2 tablespoons coconut oil
- 1 small yellow onion, halved and sliced
- 2 cloves garlic, smashed
- 1 red bell pepper, sliced
- 1 green bell pepper, sliced
- 1 small jalapeno, minced (omit seeds if you don't like spice)
- 2 pounds free-range chicken cutlets
- 1 teaspoon cumin
- 1/4 cup fresh cilantro, minced
- 1 small lime cut into wedges

Instructions

1. Heat the oil in cast-iron skillet.
2. Add the onions, and sauté for five minutes.
3. Add the garlic, and cook one more minute.
4. Add the peppers, and sauté for five minutes.
5. Remove the veggies from skillet, and place them in large bowl, and then cover them with foil.
6. Add the chicken to skillet, and sauté until cooked (about eight to ten minutes).
7. Add the veggies back into skillet.
8. Stir in the cumin, sprinkle the cilantro on top, and then turn off the heat.
9. Serve with lime wedges as garnish.
10. Enjoy with freshly steamed kale rather than rice.

DINNER

Chicken Broccoli Alfredo

Ingredients
- 1 spaghetti squash
- 2 teaspoons ghee
- 1 pound boneless, skinless chicken breasts or thighs, cut into 1-inch pieces
- 1 medium-size head of broccoli, chopped
- 2 cloves of garlic, minced
- sea salt and pepper to taste
- 2 tablespoons grass-fed butter
- 1 tablespoon coconut flour
- 1 cup unsweetened almond milk
- pinch of nutmeg

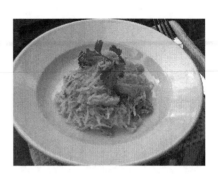

Instructions
1. Preheat the oven to 375 degrees Fahrenheit.
2. Cut the spaghetti squash in half lengthwise, and scoop out the seeds with a spoon. Place it skin side up in a baking pan, and fill the pan about 1/4 inch high with water. Place the pan in the oven, and bake the squash for thirty minutes.
3. Now, whip up the sauce. Melt the grass-fed butter in a small saucepan over medium heat, and then whisk in the coconut flour to make a roux. Whisk constantly for a couple minutes, and then slowly add the almond milk. Continue to whisk the mixture for five minutes or until it has thickened. Add the nutmeg, and season to taste with sea salt and pepper. Set this aside.
4. Heat the ghee in a large pan over medium heat. Add the garlic, and sauté it briefly. Add the chicken pieces,and season with sea salt and pepper. Let this cook for a few minutes, stirring occasionally. Next add the broccoli pieces, and sauté it with the chicken. Turn the heat down to medium-low, and continue to stir occasionally until the chicken is done and the broccoli is tender. Once done, keep it warm over low heat.

5. Once the spaghetti squash is done and cool enough to handle, scrape out the shreds (noodles) with a fork. Add the noodles to the pan with the chicken and broccoli, and then pour the sauce over top. Mix together over low heat until well incorporated. Add more sea salt and pepper if necessary.

Lemon Garlic Herb Pork Chops

Instructions

4 *bone-in* pork chops
3 tablespoons olive oil
zest from one lemon
juice from one lemon
2 to 3 cloves garlic, *minced*
1 tablespoon dried thyme
1 tablespoon dried basil
1/2 tablespoon crushed black pepper
1 teaspoon sea salt *flakes*

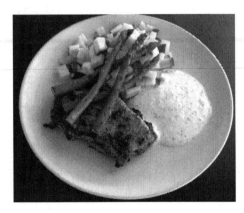

Instructions

Make three to four cuts through the fat cap of each pork chop, and put them in a large plastic bag.

Mix the rest of the ingredients in a bowl, and then pour it into the bag with the pork chops.

Try to get the air out of the bag and seal it with as little air as possible but still space for the pork chops to move around a bit.

Start massaging the bag until the pork chops are evenly rubbed and covered with the marinade.

Place them in the fridge for at least a few hours before grilling them over direct heat.

(Take them out of the fridge when you light the grill so that they are room temperature when you start to grill them.)
Serve with grilled asparagus and zucchini lightly salted.

Zucchini and Ground Beef

Ingredients

- 1 tablespoon coconut oil
- 1/2 yellow onion, diced
- 1 pound lean ground beef
- 1 to 2 cloves garlic, minced
- 2 tablespoons dried oregano
- 2 medium (6- to 8-inch) zucchinis, diced
- 2 medium tomatoes, diced
- 1/2 teaspoon sea salt (optional)

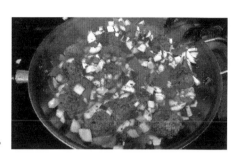

Instructions

1. Wash and prepare the vegetables.
2. Heat a large skillet over medium-high heat. Add the coconut oil when hot.
3. Add the onions to the skillet, and sauté them until they are slightly translucent.
4. Quickly roll the ground beef into balls, and add them to the pan, along with the garlic and oregano. Cook for five minutes, stirring occasionally.
5. Add the zucchini and tomatoes, and cook until tender.
6. Season with sea salt if desired.

Hatch Chile Meatballs

Ingredients

1 pound grass-fed ground beef

1/2 Hatch chile, minced

1/2 jalapeno, minced

1 teaspoon cumin

1 teaspoon paprika

1 teaspoon salt

2 tablespoons cilantro, minced

2 tablespoons onion, minced

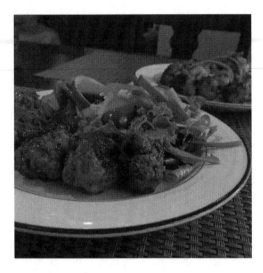

Instructions

In a mixing bowl, gently combine all the ingredients with your hands. You don't want to over-work the meat. Gently roll the mixture in to twelve evenly sized meatballs. Cook these over medium-high heat in your cast-iron skillet for about fifteen minutes or until medium, flipping them halfway through.

∎Herb Spinach Chicken Burgers

Ingredients

- 1 pound ground chicken
- 1/4 cup fresh parsley, roughly chopped
- 1 1/2 cups fresh spinach, roughly chopped
- 1/2 yellow onion, diced
- 1 garlic clove, minced
- 2 teaspoons dried thyme
- 1 teaspoon dried basil
- 1 teaspoon garlic powder
- sliced avocado (to garnish)
- salt and pepper to taste
- 1 large yellow onion, thinly sliced
- 2 tablespoons coconut oil
- 1 tablespoon water
- pinch of salt

Instructions

1. Place a medium saucepan over medium heat, along with the fat of choice and sliced onions for your caramelized onions.
2. Let the onions begin to cook down, moving them around at times to make sure they don't stick to the bottom. When the onions begin to brown slightly, pour in a tablespoon of water to help steam and cook the onions.
3. While the onions cook down, put all the ingredients for your burgers into a large bowl, and use your hands to mix well.
4. Form five balls with your hands.

5. Place a nonstick large skillet over medium heat. Once the skillet is hot, place a couple of your balls of meat onto the skillet, and then press down with a spatula to flatten them out.
6. Cook them on both sides for six to eight minutes. I flipped mine a couple times to make sure they didn't burn but browned up nicely.
7. Once the burgers are done cooking, top them with the onions and avocado.

◼Simple Bacon and Spinach–Stuffed Chicken

Ingredients

- 4 chicken breasts, butterflied and pounded flat
- 6 to 8 ounces button mushrooms, roughly chopped
- 5 strips of bacon
- 4 to 5 cups fresh spinach
- 2 garlic cloves, minced
- salt and pepper to taste

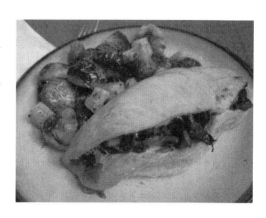

Instructions

1. Preheat the oven to 350 degrees Fahrenheit.
2. Butterfly your chicken. I'm not totally sure how to butterfly a chicken breast, but I cut mine in half. Then place plastic wrap on top of the chicken, and pound it until it is flat.
3. Then place a large skillet on medium-high heat.
4. Add the five strips of bacon, cook it on both sides until crispy, and then place the bacon on a paper towel to soak up the excess fat. When cooled, dice up the bacon.
5. Pour out the excess fat from the bacon, leaving behind about 3 tablespoons in the pan.
6. While the pan is still over medium-high heat, toss in the garlic cloves, and then add diced mushrooms.
7. Sprinkle in a bit of salt and pepper on the mushrooms.
8. Once the mushrooms have begun to soften, add the spinach and a bit more salt and pepper.
9. Cover and let this steam until the spinach has begun to wilt. When the spinach has wilted, remove the pan from the heat, and add in the diced bacon. Mix with the mushrooms and spinach until well combined.

10. Place the mixture into the middle of your butterflied chicken. Fold the chicken over to make a little pocket, and use two toothpicks to keep it closed while cooking.
11. Place the stuffed chicken breasts on a parchment-lined baking sheet, and put it in the oven to bake for 18 to 20 minutes or until there is no longer any pink in the chicken. The time will vary depending on how thin you pound the chicken. It may take a bit longer.

◼Easy Chicken Dinner 1...2...3...

Ingredients

- 3 to 4 chicken thighs or breasts
- 5 to 6 heads broccoli, chopped into florets
- 4 to 5 tablespoons olive oil
- 2 to 3 tablespoons balsamic vinegar
- 1 teaspoon garlic powder
- salt and pepper to taste

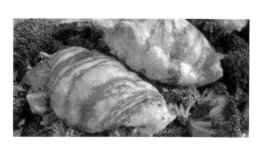

Instructions

1. Preheat the oven to 375 degrees Fahrenheit. Place the broccoli florets and chicken pieces into a 9-by-13-inch baking dish.
2. Pour olive oil and balsamic vinegar over your chicken and broccoli. Then season it with garlic powder, salt, and pepper. Mix it around to help coat the broccoli and chicken.
3. Bake it for twenty to twenty-five minutes or until the chicken is cooked through. Not sure if it's totally cooked through? Cut it open, and look.

▪Grilled Salmon with Avocado Salsa

Ingredients
2 pounds salmon cut into 4 pieces
1 tablespoon olive oil
1 teaspoon salt
1 teaspoon ground coriander
1 teaspoon ground cumin
1 teaspoon paprika powder
1 teaspoon onion powder
1 teaspoon black pepper

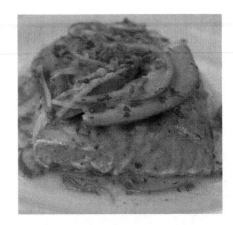

Avocado Salsa
1 avocado, peeled, seeded, and sliced
1 small red onion, sliced
3 mild hot peppers, seeded, deveined, and diced or sliced
juice from 2 limes
3 tablespoons olive oil
2 tablespoons finely chopped cilantro
salt to taste

Instructions
1. Mix the salt, coriander, cumin, paprika, onion, and black pepper together. Rub the salmon fillets with olive oil and the seasoning mix, and
   refrigerate it for at least thirty minutes.
2. Preheat the grill.
3. Combine the avocado, onion, hot peppers, cilantro, lime juice, olive oil,
   and salt in a bowl, mix well, and then chill until ready to use.
4. Grill the salmon to desired doneness.
5. Serve the salmon topped with the avocado salsa.

■Grilled Chicken with Greek Sweet Potatoes

Ingredients

- 1 chicken breast, sliced lengthwise
- 2 lemons, juiced
- 1 tablespoon dried oregano
- 2 sweet potatoes cut into large chunks
- salt and pepper
- 2 bell peppers, sliced finely
- 1/2 red onion, sliced finely
- 1/2 cup parsley, chopped roughly
- 1 cup cherry tomatoes, halved
- 1 teaspoon olive oil
- 1 clove of garlic, minced

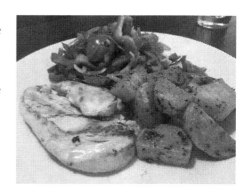

Instructions

1. Preheat the oven to 350 degrees.
2. Mix the juice of one lemon, the oregano, salt, and pepper together in a bowl, and coat the sweet potatoes.
3. Place the sweet potatoes on an oven tray, and roast them in the oven for twenty minutes. After fifteen minutes, turn the sweet potatoes over, and squeeze the juice of one half of a lemon over them.
4. While the sweet potatoes are roasting, mix the peppers, red onion, parsley, and cherry tomatoes in a bowl.
5. In a small bowl, whisk the juice of half a lemon, olive oil, and minced garlic together, and then add this to the salad, mixing it thoroughly. The salad is done.
6. Grill the chicken—the first side will need four to five minutes—then turn it over, and cook it for three to four minutes.
7. Serve the chicken breast with some sweet potatoes and the salad.

▪Simple Herb-Crusted Salmon

Ingredients
- 2 salmon fillets (6 ounces each)
- 1 heaping tablespoon coconut flour
- 2 tablespoons fresh parsley
- 1 tablespoon olive oil
- 1 tablespoon Dijon mustard
- salt and pepper to taste

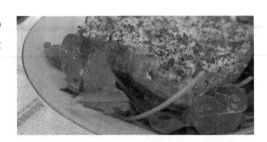

Salad
- 2 cups arugula
- 1/4 red onion, sliced thin
- juice of 1 lemon
- 1 tablespoon white-wine vinegar
- 1 tablespoon olive oil
- salt and pepper to taste

Instructions
1. Preheat the oven to 450 degrees Fahrenheit.
2. Place the salmon fillets on a parchment- or foil-lined baking sheet.
3. Top your salmon off with olive oil and Dijon mustard, and rub it into your salmon.
4. In a small bowl, mix together the coconut flour, parsley, salt, and pepper.
5. Use a spoon to sprinkle your toppings onto your salmon and then your hand to pat it into your salmon.
6. Place the salmon in the oven for ten to fifteen minutes or until it is cooked to your preference. I cook mine more on the medium-rare side at twelve minutes.
7. While the salmon is cooking, mix together your salad ingredients.
8. When the salmon is done, place it on top of salad.

◼Roasted Garlic, Spinach, and Mushroom–Stuffed Pork Chops

Ingredients

4 pieces, thick-cut, bone-in pork chops
1 head roasted garlic
2 tablespoons Dijon mustard
8 ounces mushrooms, chopped
2 cups baby spinach, chopped
salt and pepper to taste
garlic powder to taste
1 1/2 cups broth (veggie or chicken)

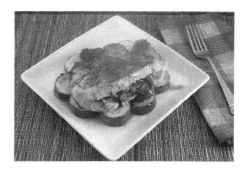

Instructions

Mix the roasted garlic and Dijon mustard together, and then set it aside. Heat 1 tablespoon of oil in a large skillet over medium-high heat. Add the chopped mushrooms, and begin to brown them. Once the mushrooms are cooked through, add the spinach. Cook it until the spinach is wilted. Add the garlic/Dijon mustard mixture, stir to combine, and heat through. Season to taste. Allow the mixture to cool before stuffing the pork chops. Starting from the side farthest from the bone, cut a slit into the pork chop until you reach the bone. (Do not cut all the way through the chop; you want a pocket to hold the stuffing). Stuff the pork chops with equal amounts of the spinach and mushroom mixture. Season the outside of the chops with salt, pepper, and garlic powder to taste.

Heat 1 tablespoon of oil in a large skillet over medium-high heat. Sear the pork chops for three to four minutes on each side (carefully turn the pork chops so that the filling doesn't fall out). Reduce the heat to medium, add the broth (scrape the browned bits off the bottom of the pan), and loosely cover. Cook for about three minutes or until the pork chops are cooked through. Remove the pork chops (keeping them warm), and reduce the sauce until thickened. Serve the sauce over the pork chops.

Pork Burgers

Ingredients

1 pound ground pork
1 teaspoon rubbed sage
1 teaspoon garlic powder
1 tablespoon Dijon mustard
1/4 to 1/2 teaspoon salt
1/4 teaspoon black pepper

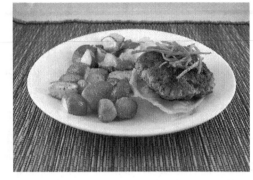

Instructions

Heat 1 tablespoon of oil in a large skillet over medium-high heat. Combine all the ingredients, and form it into four even patties. Place the patties in the skillet, and sear them for four to five minutes. Flip the patties over, and sear for another four to five minutes or until the burger is cooked through (160 Fahrenheit). Top with roasted, shredded carrots.

Chicken Piccata

Ingredients

2 pounds boneless, skinless chicken breast
1 1/2 cups chicken stock, divided
juice of 3 lemons, divided
1 clove garlic, minced
3 tablespoons capers

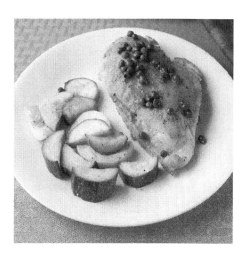

Instructions

Heat 1 to 2 tablespoons of oil in a large skillet over medium-high heat. Season the chicken with salt, pepper, and garlic powder to taste. Sear the chicken for three to four minutes per side. Add 1 cup of the chicken stock (scraping the browned bits off the bottom of the pan), juice of 2 lemons, and the garlic. Reduce the heat to medium, cover, and cook for five to seven minutes or until the chicken is cooked through. Add the remaining chicken stock, lemon juice, and the capers. Cook for one to two minutes. Serve the sauce over the chicken.

Zucchini Fettuccine Alfredo

Ingredients

- 3 to 4 organic garlic cloves
- 1 organic leek leaf
- 1 organic shallot
- 1 to 2 cups organic shiitake mushrooms (or mushrooms of your choice)
- a handful organic cilantro
- 1 tablespoon organic white chia seed powder or flaxseed meal
- 6 tablespoons organic coconut cream
- 4 tablespoons natural coconut water
- 3 tablespoons organic coconut oil (1 tablespoon for frying)
- 1 happy free-range egg yolk
- sea salt to taste
- organic black pepper to taste
- 2 zucchinis

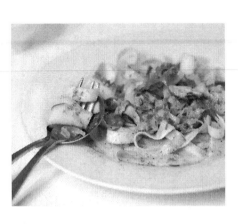

Instructions

1. On a cutting board, chop the garlic, leek, and shallots. Set these aside for five to ten minutes.
2. Chop the mushrooms, and set them aside.
3. In a frying pan, add the coconut oil at low-medium heat.
4. Lightly fry the garlic, leeks, shallots, and mushrooms for about three minutes. Set this aside.
5. Chop the cilantro, and put it in a mixing bowl.
6. Add flaxseed meal, coconut cream, coconut water, coconut oil, and the egg yolk to the mixing bowl. Add the mushroom mixture, and combine well. The subtle heat from the mushrooms and onions will help mix everything into a sauce-like texture. Set this aside. (You have the option of heating the sauce after you mix it; I chose not to so that the zucchini pasta stays cold with live enzymes.)

7. Using a carrot peeler, peel the zucchini lengthwise (until you reach the seeds).
8. Evenly distribute the peels, including the skins, to two plates. Do not discard the skin peels, as they hold the most nutrition.
9. Top off the pasta with the alfredo sauce.

Crispy-Skin Salmon

Ingredients

- 1 1/2 pound salmon fillet, skin on
- 2 cloves garlic
- 3 sprigs fresh thyme
- salt and pepper to taste
- 1 tablespoon olive oil

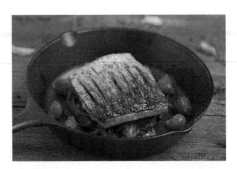

Instructions

1. Take the salmon fillet, and cut it into individual portions according to how much each person eats.

2. Flip the salmon over, skin side up, firmly hold the sides of the fillet while curling it upward by pressing the sides slightly in. Carefully score the skin across by slicing your knife through the skin about half an inch deep. Be sure to do this just across the top of the skin, but do not slice all the way through the fish like you are going to cut it in half. Try to keep the scores about a quarter of an inch apart; the closer the scores the crispier the skin.

3. Once each fillet is scored, take the leaves off your thyme, and mince them with your garlic.

4. Sprinkle in a little bit of salt, freshly cracked black pepper, and thyme-garlic mixture in between each slit of each score.

5. In a medium-size pan, heat the oil over medium-high heat, and wait for the pan to get hot. While you're waiting for the pan to get hot, lightly brush the top of each salmon skin with oil to prevent sticking. (Be careful not to rub out any of the herb mixture from the slits.)

6. Once the pan is hot, place the salmon in the pan, facing away from you so as not to splash hot oil on yourself, and very lightly press down for a second to make sure it's evenly distributed across the pan for an even sear. (Take care not to overcrowd the pan, as you may need to do the salmon in batches.)

7. Let the salmon cook for two to four minutes on the skin or until it has turned a milky pink about two-thirds the way up the salmon.
8. Carefully slide a spatula or fish fry under the salmon (be careful not to rip the skin), and flip and cook the other side for two to three more minutes or until the salmon is cooked all the way through.
9. Serve with your choice of veggies. I like mine served with charred grape tomatoes and sautéed spinach.

SNACKS

HEALTHY SNACKING

In between meals, you have the option of snacking. Healthy snacking is suggested to maintain good metabolism and will also give you energy throughout the day. Healthy snacking is also a good idea if you are out and about all day and can't get a full meal in. It will hold you over until your next meal and prevent you from getting too hungry. However, the wrong approach to snacks can certainly harm even the best diet.

Following are lists of healthy snacks that can be bought or made for snacking in between meals. These ideas should help you avoid reaching for unhealthy snacks (which shouldn't be in your home in the first place).

Snacks to Have on Hand
 Nuts
- Almonds
- Cashews
- Macadamia
- Walnuts
- Chestnuts
- Hazelnuts
- Pistachios
- Pine nuts
- Pecans

 Seeds
- Pumpkin
- Sunflower
- Flax

If you can find store-bought jerky with no sugar or soy sauce, it's a great snack option; otherwise, you can make your own in a dehydrator or even in the oven. Beef is traditional, but buffalo and turkey jerky are also tasty.

If you chop up some carrot or celery sticks and toss them into plastic bags in the fridge, you'll have an easy snack to grab and go with all week.

Make Your Own

Hard-boiled eggs: Eggs aren't just a breakfast food. Hard-boiled eggs are simple to make and travel well for a protein boost on the go.

Roasted pumpkin seeds: You can buy these or just scoop out the seeds when you cook a pumpkin. Roast them in some coconut oil with a dash of sea salt until they're a light golden-brown.

Crispy kale chips: Cut the stems out of several kale leaves, sprinkle with olive oil and sea salt, and bake at 275 degrees Fahrenheit for forty minutes, turning them over halfway through.

Slices of deli meat: Turkey, roast-beef, or ham slices can be easily stored in a small bag or container.

Cucumber cups: Cut a cucumber into slices about two inches thick, hollow out the centers, and stuff them with tuna or salmon. These are perfect finger foods for a party since they're not messy to eat.

Guacamole with veggies: Guacamole is a wonderful snack full of healthy fats and vitamins. Try it with peppers or carrots for added crunch.

Cucumber sandwiches: A small piece of meat between two crunchy cucumber slices makes a refreshing bite on the run.

Sweet-potato fries: Cut a sweet potato into French fry–size pieces, toss with coconut oil, sprinkle with sea salt, and bake on a cookie tray for about twenty to twenty-five minutes.

Chili Lime Jicama Sticks

Ingredients
- 2 pounds jicama, peeled and cut into 1/4-inch sticks
- 1/4 lime juice from 1 lime
- 1 tablespoon chopped fresh cilantro
- 1/4 teaspoon red-pepper flakes
- fine sea salt to taste
- freshly ground black pepper to taste
- chipotle powder to taste

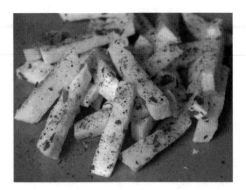

Instructions
Combine the jicama, lime juice, cilantro, and red-pepper flakes in a large bowl, and toss until well incorporated. Place the dressed jicama on a large platter, and season it with salt, pepper, and chipotle powder. Serve immediately.

Crunchy Roasted Chickpeas

Ingredients

2 cans chickpeas
3 tablespoons extra-virgin olive oil
coarse sea salt
1 1/2 teaspoons cinnamon, paprika,
pepper, etc. (optional)

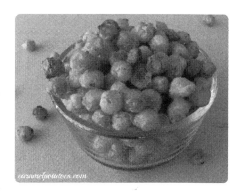

Instructions

Preheat the oven to 400 degrees
Fahrenheit. Drain and rinse the
chickpeas, and scatter them on a
rimmed baking sheet lined with paper towels. Let this stand for fifteen minutes. Remove the paper towels, and toss the chickpeas with olive oil.

Roast the chickpeas until crisp and golden, about forty-five minutes, stirring occasionally. Toss with coarse salt and 1 1/2 teaspoons of desired seasoning before serving. Store cooled chickpeas in an airtight container for up to one week.

Paleo Spiced Nuts

Ingredients
- 2/3 cup almonds
- 2/3 cup pecans
- 2/3 cup walnuts
- 1 teaspoon chili powder
- 1/2 teaspoon cumin
- 1/2 teaspoon black pepper
- 1/2 teaspoon Celtic sea salt
- 1 tablespoon olive oil

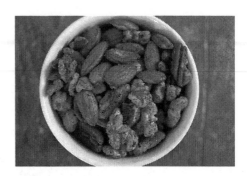

Instructions
1. Place the nuts in a large cast-iron skillet over medium heat. Toast them until lightly browned.
2. While the nuts are toasting, prepare the spice mixture.
3. Combine chili, cumin, black pepper, and salt in a small bowl.
4. Coat the nuts with olive oil, and then coat them with the spice mixture, and serve

Roasted Pumpkin Seeds with a Twist

Ingredients

2 cups pumpkin seeds, washed

4 teaspoons olive oil

2 teaspoons garlic salt

2 teaspoons onion powder

1 teaspoon hot sauce

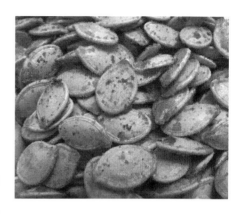

Instructions

Preheat the oven to 300 degrees Fahrenheit.

Place the seeds in a bowl, and add olive oil and the seasonings.

Mix well.

Spread the pumpkin seeds in a single layer on a baking sheet.

Bake for about thirty minutes, depending on your oven. Stir halfway through baking.

✎ Zucchini Chips

Ingredients
2 zucchinis
1 teaspoon of olive oil
1/4 teaspoon of salt
1/4 to 1/2 teaspoon of garlic powder
ground pepper to taste

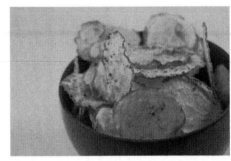

Instructions
1. Slice two medium zucchinis (about 1/2 pound each) thinly with a mandolin.
2. Toss the sliced zucchinis in a bowl with olive oil, salt, and garlic powder.
3. Line the dehydrator screen with the zucchinis, without the flex sheets or parchment to allow them to dry better (a common problem with dehydrating the zucchinis seems to be getting them crispy dry).
4. Sprinkle them with freshly ground pepper.
5. Dehydrate at 140 degrees Fahrenheit for about four hours or until dry and crispy.

DESSERTS

Strawberry Ice Cream

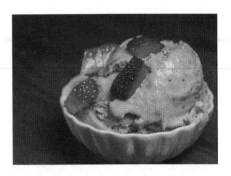

Ingredients

28 ounces organic, full-fat coconut milk
(2 cans)
1 tablespoon vanilla extract
2 pastured eggs
3 tablespoons coconut nectar or raw
honey
2 to 2 1/2 cups organic strawberries
(stems removed)
3 teaspoons of freshly squeezed lemon juice (from an organic lemon)
dash of sea salt

Instructions

In a medium saucepan, heat the coconut milk on low-medium heat (do not boil it).

Add the vanilla extract, coconut nectar (or honey), lemon juice, and sea salt, whisking it to incorporate everything.

Remove the mixture from the heat.

In a small bowl, beat the eggs, and then add them to the coconut-milk mixture, whisking constantly until the eggs are fully incorporated (about two minutes).

Wash the strawberries, remove the stems, and then puree them in a blender or food processor.

Add the pureed strawberries to the coconut milk, and stir it to incorporate.

Let the mixture cool to room temperature.

When the mixture is cool (I put mine in the refrigerator to chill), add it to your ice-cream maker, and follow the manufacturer's instructions.

If you don't have an ice-cream maker, pour the mixture into a glass bowl or 9-by-12-inch Pyrex pan, and place it in your freezer. Stir the ice cream mixture every ten to fifteen minutes until it reaches your desired consistency. This ice cream can be made vegan by eliminating the eggs and using coconut nectar or your favorite vegan sweetener.

This ice cream is not overly sweet, so add more coconut nectar, honey, or a little stevia to sweeten to your liking.

Coconut Crème Brûlée

Ingredients
- 1/3 cup extra creamy coconut milk
- 3 egg yolks
- 3 tablespoons + 8 teaspoons coconut palm sugar
- 1 vanilla bean
- 2 tablespoons shredded coconut, divided

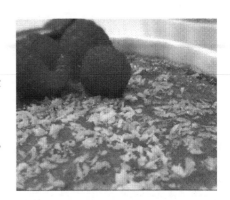

Instructions
Preheat the oven to 320 degrees Fahrenheit.

Set a kettle of water to boil.

Place four crème brûlée dishes in a deep baking pan.

Put the coconut milk in a pot.

With a knife, split the vanilla bean lengthwise, and scrape out the seeds using the backside of the blade.

Add the seeds and the scraped out pod to the coconut milk.

Slowly bring it to a boil over low heat, and then set it aside.

In a bowl, whisk the egg yolks and the 3 tablespoons of coconut sugar.

Remove the vanilla pod from the coconut milk, and then slowly pour it into the egg yolk and coconut sugar mix while rapidly whisking.

Using a ladle, divide equally into the crème brûlée dishes, and stir between each scoop to get the vanilla seeds evenly distributed. Fill the dishes almost all the way up to the rim.

Pour the hot water into the baking pan so that it reaches at least halfway up the outside of the crème brûlée dishes.

Carefully transfer the baking pan to the oven. (You do not want waves of water splashing into the crème brûlée.)

Bake them for forty-five minutes, and then, just as carefully, take the pan out of the oven.

Transfer the crème brûlée dishes to another tray with a wide but sturdy spatula.

Let them cool down a bit, cover them with plastic wrap, and place the tray in the fridge for at least a few hours.

Take the tray from the fridge.

Turn on the oven broiler.

In a dry frying pan, roast 1 tablespoon of shredded coconut until it turns light brown.

Sprinkle 1 teaspoon of coconut palm sugar evenly over each crème brûlée, and then sprinkle the roasted coconut on top of that.

Run them under the broiler for about three minutes.

Sprinkle another teaspoon of coconut palm sugar over each, then run for another three minutes under the broiler.

Take them out, sprinkle some shredded (not roasted) coconut over the tops, and let them cool down in the fridge for about five to ten minutes.

You don't want to serve them hot, but slightly warm is perfectly OK and definitely better than cold.

Serve as is or garnish with some fresh berries if you like.

Berry Parfait

Ingredients
- 1 pint blueberries
- 2 large handfuls strawberries
- 2 bunches red seedless grapes
- 1 1/4 cups blanched almond flour
- 1/3 cup water
- 1/2 teaspoon Celtic sea salt
- 1 teaspoon apple-cider vinegar
- 1 teaspoon lemon juice
- 1 heaping tablespoon raw honey
- few drops vanilla

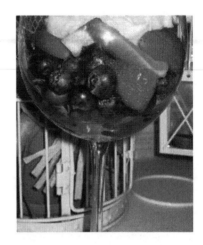

Instructions
In place of whipped cream or yogurt, this recipe uses a sweet almond flour-based cream cheese. The cream cheese can be made ahead of time and chilled in the refrigerator (it is best served cold).

1. Create your sweet cream cheese by blending all ingredients *except* the berries and grapes in a blender or food processor until thick and creamy. Chill this in the refrigerator (or freezer if you have less time).
2. Wash and dry all your berries. Hull and slice the strawberries, but leave the blueberries and grapes whole.
3. Arrange a few handfuls of grapes and blueberries in the bottom of a large wine goblet. Top these with the sliced strawberries.
4. Usa a few dollops of sweet almond cream cheese over all of it. Take care not to use too much, as it will overwhelm the fruit in the glass. About two heaping spoonfuls should be plenty.

Paleo Brownies

Ingredients

2 eggs

1/2 teaspoon vanilla

6 tablespoons oil (I usually use 3 tablespoons apple sauce and 3 tablespoons coconut cream/ oil)

1/2 cup (or to taste) of honey

1/2 cup almond flour

1/2 cup unsweetened cocoa

1/4 cup arrowroot

chopped nuts

chopped up bits of unsweetened cooking chocolate

Instructions

1. Beat the egg whites until they form stiff peaks in a bowl (you can use whole eggs if you're happy with denser brownies).
2. In another bowl, beat the egg yolks, and then add and mix in all the other ingredients.
3. Fold in the egg whites.
4. Bake at 350 degrees Fahrenheit for about thirty minutes.

Coconut Truffle

Ingredients

- 1 can good-quality coconut milk (full fat)
- 3 tablespoons raw honey
- 1/2 cup shredded coconut (unsweetened)
- 1 tablespoon butter
- 1/2 teaspoon vanilla extract

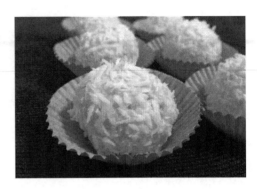

Instructions

Mix the coconut milk and the honey in a saucepan.

Bring it to a boil, and then simmer it for about two hours, stirring the mixture once in a while.

You will notice the mixture getting thicker, and after two hours, it should be thick enough so that it does not run off the spoon easily. Add the butter and the shredded coconut, and cook it for about five minutes, stirring constantly so it does not burn. When the mixture starts to release off the bottom of the pan and has a very thick consistency, remove it from the stove, and let it cool. Place the mixture in the fridge for about two hours. It is important that it is cool before you roll it.

Remove it from fridge, grease your hands with butter, and start rolling the truffles into balls, and then roll each ball in the shredded coconut.

EATING OUT

Tips

Here are some tips for eating out and sticking as closely as possible to the Diet Plan.

- First off, pick a restaurant that uses fresh ingredients. They're often the ones who source local, organic, grass-fed, pastured products and know their menus and ingredients inside out.
- Get a salad, and order extra meat or hard-boiled eggs if your meal doesn't already come with enough protein. Ask for olive oil and vinegar as dressing.
- Order a burger—no bun— and a salad with a side of guacamole or plain avocado.
- Order a meat, chicken, or fish entrée with extra veggies.

So if you're being as strict as possible, ask these kinds of questions of your waitstaff:

- What kind of oil is [enter menu item here] sautéed in?
- Is the chicken (or any other meat) battered in flour?
- Is there milk, butter, or cheese in that?

Tip on Cuisine
At a Steak House
Think meat and veggies. Instead of a starchy side, just order an extra-large portion of veggies and a salad with oil, vinegar, and lemon. Don't forget to ask for a burger without the bun (add bacon and avocado).

At a Mexican Restaurant
Think fajita bowl! Get two kinds of meat, say chicken and steak, and add guacamole, salsa, and jalapenos. You can also ask to turn any burrito into a bowl, and just say no rice and beans.

At a Chinese/Mandarin Restaurant

Order without noodles or rice, and nothing fried. Just meat and veggie stir-fry.

At a Thai Restaurant

Tom Gha soup is the absolute best. Just mushrooms, chicken, coconut milk, and lime. They also typically have really good meat and veggie dishes. Curry is also a must, but without the rice.

At an Italian Restaurant

Chicken picatta, not breaded, is a great choice; just make sure you ask them if they bread it first. A lot of times, you can substitute a plain chicken breast. Chicken simmered in butter and wine with capers without pasta is another good option. Make sure to order a veggie or salad side. You can also keep your eyes out for meatballs and marinara without pasta. It's good to ask if they use sugar in their marinara as well.

At a Breakfast Joint

Go nuts here. Eggs, bacon, ham, and a side of avocado. If you're having coffee, try to use whole or almond milk; if they have coconut milk, you know you've found your breakfast heaven!

At a Sushi Restaurant

Go for the sashimi, or ask for your rolls without rice. Order hand rolls with fish and veggies but no rice.

EXTRAS
AND
ALTERNATIVES

Asparagus Basil Salad

Ingredients

1 pound asparagus, trimmed and halved

1 cup grape tomatoes, halved

1 ripe avocado, cut into cubes

1 cup sliced basil leaves

1/4 cup olive oil

2 teaspoons lemon juice

2 teaspoons Dijon mustard

1/2 teaspoon Celtic sea salt

1/2 teaspoon pepper

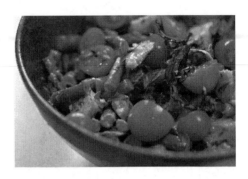

Instructions

1. Steam the asparagus for five to seven minutes until tender.
2. Place the asparagus, tomatoes, avocado, and basil in a large bowl.
3. Stir in the olive oil, lemon juice, and mustard.
4. Sprinkle with salt and pepper.

Dijon Pork–Stuffed Zucchini

Ingredients

5 medium zucchinis
1 pound ground pork
1 teaspoon rubbed sage
1 teaspoon fennel (optional to grind the seeds to form a powder)
1 teaspoon garlic powder
1/2 teaspoon salt
1/2 teaspoon pepper
2 tablespoons Dijon mustard

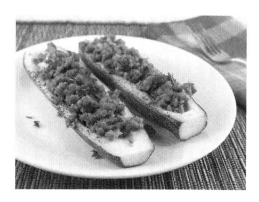

Instructions

Preheat the oven to 350 degrees Fahrenheit. Cut the ends off of the zucchini, and cut each zucchini in half. Using a spoon, remove the core/seeds from the zucchini, and chop it into small pieces. Set this aside for later. Place the zucchini in a baking dish. Heat a large skillet over medium-high heat. Add the ground pork, and begin to brown it. Add the spices, and continue to brown the pork until cooked through. Add the reserved zucchini core/seeds, and cook for another one to two minutes. Add the Dijon mustard, and heat through.

Sprinkle the zucchini with salt and pepper to taste. Fill the zucchini with the pork mixture. Bake uncovered for twenty-five to thirty minutes or until the zucchinis are tender.

Garlic Grilled Tomatoes

Ingredients
- tomatoes
- garlic
- olive oil
- herbs

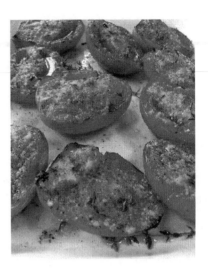

Instructions
1. Crush garlic, oil, and herbs in a small bowl.
2. Slice the tomatoes in half, and brush them with the garlic-oil-herb mix.
3. Throw them into a frying pan or grill them until slightly burned.

▪Ginger Lime Kale with Squash and Chickpeas

Ingredients

- 2 cups chopped butternut squash, peeled and seeded (cut into 3/4-inch cubes)
- 1 1/2 tablespoons olive oil, divided
- 1 medium onion, diced
- 2 cloves garlic, minced
- 1 tablespoon freshly grated ginger root
- 8 cups thinly sliced kale leaves
- 1 1/2 cups organic canned chickpeas, drained and rinsed
- 1 tablespoon fresh lime juice
- 1/4 teaspoon sea salt
- 1/2 cup fresh pomegranate arils

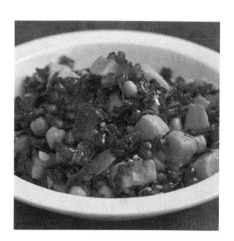

Instructions

1. Preheat the oven to 400 degrees Fahrenheit. In a medium bowl, toss the squash with a 1/2 tablespoon of oil. Spread the squash onto a parchment-lined, rimmed baking sheet, and roast it for about twenty-five minutes or until the squash is tender and lightly browned. Remove the squash from the oven, and let it cool.

2. Heat a wide and deep skillet over low-medium heat. Add the remaining 1 tablespoon of oil to coat the skillet. Add the onion, and cook it, stirring constantly, for five minutes. Add the garlic and ginger, stirring for thirty seconds. Add the kale, stirring for one minute until the kale begins to wilt. Reduce the heat to low, cover, and cook for ten minutes, stirring once or twice. Add the chickpeas, and stir again. Cover and cook it for another five minutes or until the chickpeas are heated through. Remove the pan from the heat, and add squash, lime juice, and salt. Transfer the mixture to a large serving bowl, and sprinkle it with pomegranate arils. Serve immediately.

🌿 ◼ No-Potato Salad

Ingredients

1 head cauliflower
2 stalks celery, diced
1 small onion, finely chopped (about
3 to 4 tablespoons)
1 tablespoon parsley, finely chopped
2 eggs, hard-boiled and diced
2 tablespoons grape-seed oil grape-
seed oil vegenaise
1 tablespoon Dijon mustard
1/2 teaspoon Celtic sea salt

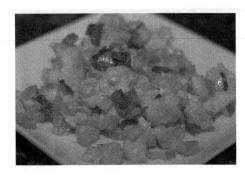

Instructions

1. Chop the cauliflower into small, 1/2-inch florets.
2. Steam the cauliflower on the stove until tender.
3. Allow the cauliflower to cool, and then place it in a large bowl.
4. Add th ecelery, onion, parsley, and eggs.
5. Stir in Vegenaise, mustard, and salt.

◢ ◼ Quinoa Mushroom Pilaf

Ingredients

olive oil

2 cloves garlic, finely chopped

1 small to medium yellow bell pepper, diced

1 small to medium green bell pepper, diced

2 cups sliced mushrooms

sea salt and ground pepper to taste

2 tablespoons freshly chopped parsley

1 teaspoon Greek seasoning (mint, lemon, basil, and oregano mix)

2 scallions (spring onions) sliced

squeeze of fresh lemon juice

olive oil to taste

2 tablespoons fresh chopped parsley

1 teaspoon Greek Seasoning (mint, lemon, basil, oregano mix)

2 scallions (spring onions) sliced-white and light green sections

Squeeze of fresh lemon juice

Extra virgin olive oil, to taste

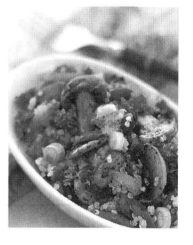

Instructions

Cook the quinoa as you normally would. When it is almost done, heat a splash of olive oil in a large skillet over medium heat. Add the garlic and yellow and green pepper, and stir it over medium heat until slightly softened. Add in the mushrooms. Season with sea salt and ground pepper to taste. Add the Greek seasoning. Stir in and cook it until the mushrooms are tender. Scoop the cooked quinoa out of the rice cooker, and add it into the mushroom-pepper mixture. Add in the sliced scallions. Stir to combine. Squeeze fresh lemon juice all over the quinoa, and drizzle it with extra-virgin olive oil. Toss well to coat the quinoa.

Taste, and add more salt or seasoning if necessary.

Sprinkle with toasted pine nuts if desired.

Serve immediately, or allow it to cool, and then cover and refrigerate it to eat as a salad.

Before serving this quinoa cold, taste it again, and adjust the seasonings. Chilling often dulls the flavors in these kinds of salads. I usually allow quinoa salad a few minutes out of the fridge before serving; letting it to come to room temperature helps the flavors. If making it ahead of time as a salad, I use water instead of broth.

Raw Zucchini, Carrot, and Cashew Salad Rolls

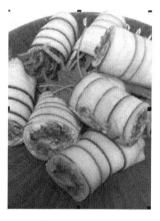

Ingredients

3 medium organic zucchinis, shaved thinly lengthwise

1/2 organic carrot, julienned or grated

1/2 organic red bell pepper, julienned or finely sliced

1 organic Lebanese cucumber, julienned or finely sliced

1/4 cup organic coriander leaves

1/4 cup organic mint leaves, roughly chopped

1 cup raw organic cashews, soaked a few hours or overnight

1/4 teaspoon sea salt

1/2 tablespoon organic lemon juice (or cider vinegar)

1/4 to 1/2 cup filtered water

1 ripe organic avocado

2 tablespoons organic red onion, finely diced

1/2 lime, juiced

dash of Tabasco to taste

Instructions

To make the salad filling, gently toss the carrots, red bell pepper, cucumber, coriander, and mint in a large bowl. You can add rocket leaves to the salad for a peppery bite.

To make the cashew sour cream, drain the cashews, place them in a food processor, add the sea salt, lemon juice, and water, and then puree everything until smooth. Refrigerate this until needed.

To assemble the rolls, lay about eight zucchini strips lengthways and close together, spread a spoonful of sour cream, guacamole, and salad on top, and then roll them up tightly. Cut into sections, and eat straight away.

✿ ▪ Roasted Rosemary Brussels and Rutabaga

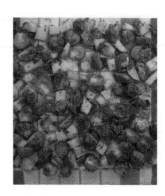

Ingredients
- 2 cups Brussels sprouts, halved
- 1 cup rutabaga, peeled and diced (I peel my rutabaga with a carrot peeler)
- 4 tablespoons fat of choice (I use olive oil)
- 1 tablespoon chopped rosemary (fresh or dried)
- salt and pepper to taste

Instructions
1. Preheat the oven to 405 degrees Fahrenheit.
2. Place the vegetables in a 9-by-13-inch glass baking dish.
3. Pour your fat of choice over the vegetables, and then toss them with rosemary, salt, and pepper.
4. Bake everything for twenty-five to thirty minutes.

More Information

If you do not cook or eat out, the following websites provide premade meals that ship directly to your door. Meals are precooked, vacuum-packed, and frozen. All you have to do is place the meal pack in water and microwave.
http://premadepaleo.com/
http://modpaleo.com/
http://www.briansbowls.com/

Or search online for paleo diet or paleo recipes.

Made in the USA
San Bernardino, CA
20 October 2015